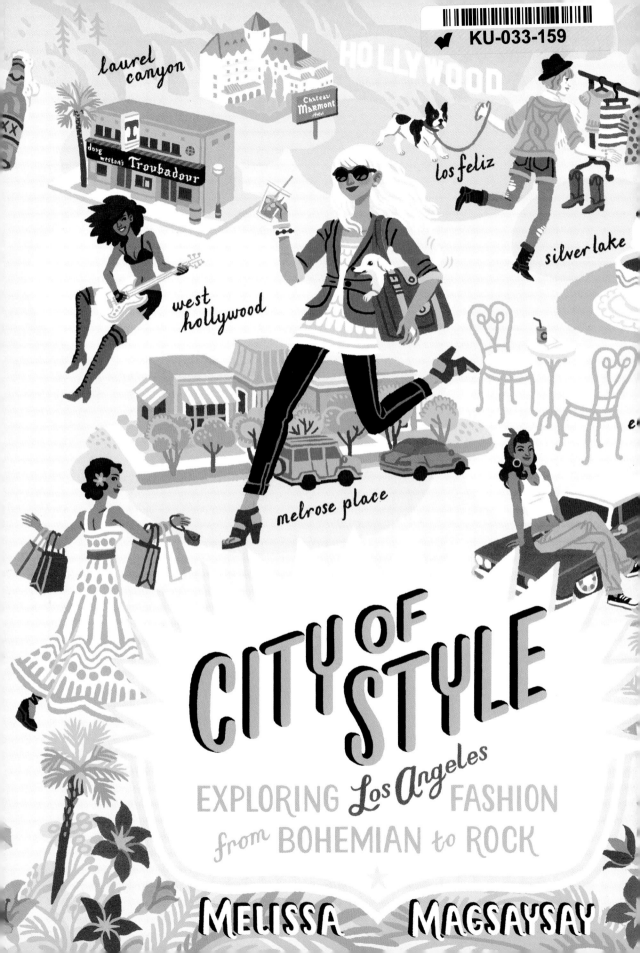

laurel canyon

Chateau Marmont Hotel

HOLLYWOOD

doug weston's Troubadour

los feliz

silver lake

west hollywood

melrose place

CITY OF STYLE

EXPLORING *Los Angeles* FASHION

from BOHEMIAN *to* ROCK

MELISSA MAGSAYSAY

HarperCollins books may be purchased for educational, business, or sales promotional use. For information please write: Special Markets Department, HarperCollins Publishers, 10 East 53rd Street, New York, NY 10022.

FIRST EDITION

Designed by Paula Russell Szafranski

Original scenic photography throughout by Donato Sardella.
Illustrations for "How to Get the Look" by Melissa Boock.
Cover and title page illustions by Kali Ciesemier.

Library of Congress Cataloging-in-Publication Data is available upon request.

ISBN 978-0-06-208840-6

12 13 14 15 16   OV/QGT   10 9 8 7 6 5 4 3 2 1

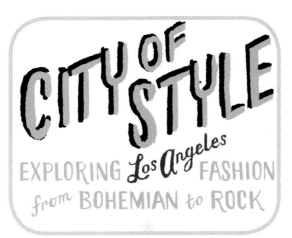

CITY OF STYLE

EXPLORING *Los Angeles* FASHION

from BOHEMIAN *to* ROCK

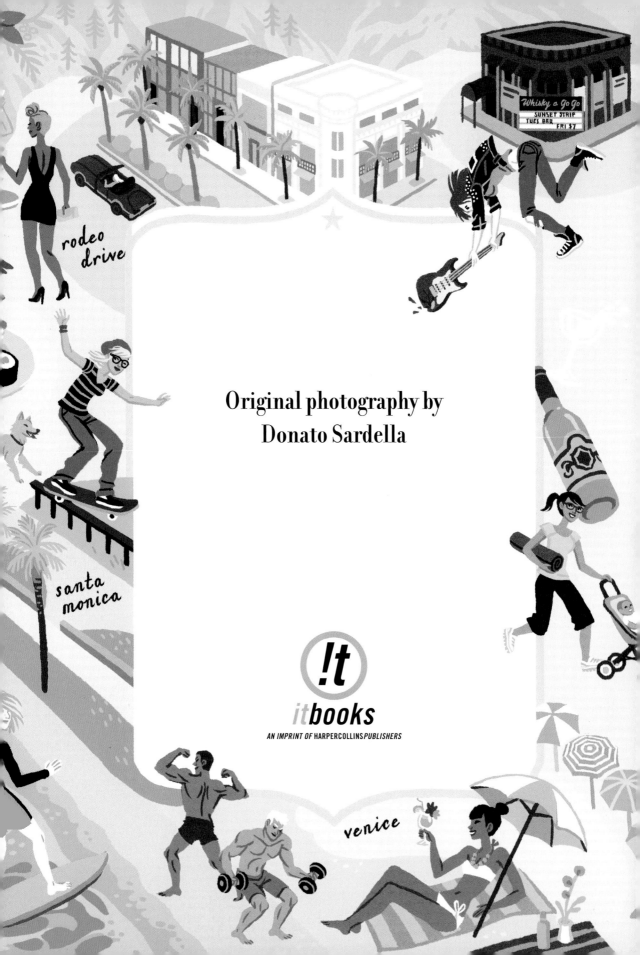

Original photography by
Donato Sardella

itbooks
AN IMPRINT OF HARPERCOLLINS PUBLISHERS

For my family

contents

FOREWORD BY AMBER VALLETTA   ix

INTRODUCTION   **xi**

ONE   Romantic Bohemians   1

TWO   Glamour   23

THREE   Skaters and Surfers   43

FOUR   Rockers   71

FIVE   Chola-Style   95

SIX   Indie Eclectic   115

SEVEN   Casual Chic   143

PHOTOGRAPHY CREDITS   **173**

ACKNOWLEDGMENTS   **178**

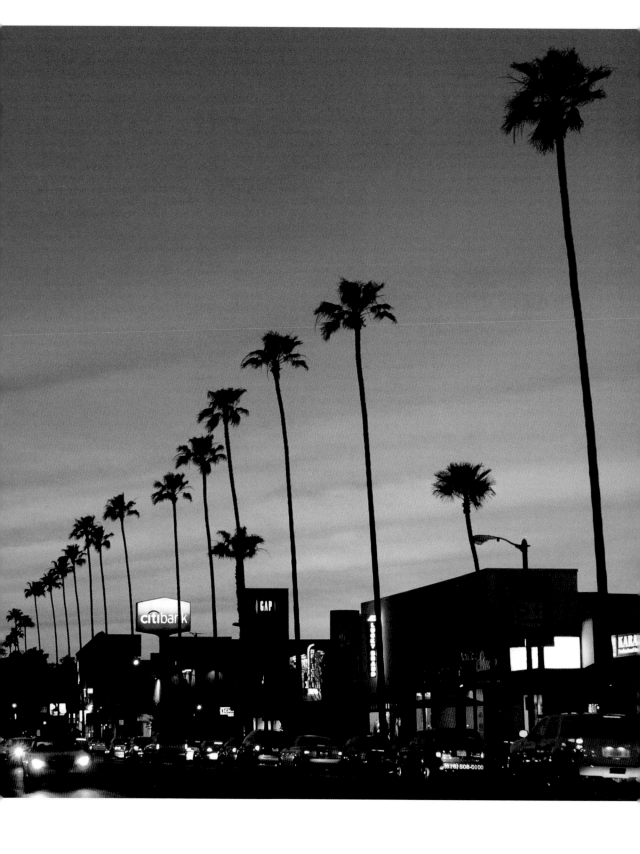

Foreword

Los Angeles isn't the easiest place to get dressed. When I was seventeen and working as a model in Milan, Paris, and New York, I wouldn't give a second thought to wearing an Alaïa cocktail dress in the middle of the day or high-waist pants, a sharp jacket, and big heels just because. But when I moved to LA to raise my son in 2001, I quickly realized that the tailored, formal pieces that worked so effortlessly in Europe and Manhattan didn't quite work the same way in perpetually sunny SoCal. And I found myself struggling to find a style that truly felt like me.

During this period of searching my style soul, I chopped off my hair and started favoring Converse sneakers, baggy jeans, and oversize button-downs in an effort to channel the old skater I had lurking inside. And that's when it hit me: My fashion sense wasn't lost. I just found a style that this town had birthed in the first place.

Los Angeles isn't just about getting dressed. It's about how you do it.

This is a rich, vibrant city, and it has created many of the most basic fashion trends that today serve as a foundation of style all over the world. Whether it's the 1970s sportswear favored by skaters and surfers, the easy-breezy bohemian dresses worn by the prolific songwriters of the 60s while they crafted melodies in our canyons, or the beaded flapper dresses that freed our earliest movie stars from the

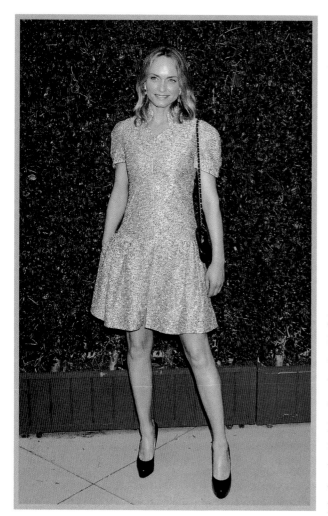

Amber Valletta attends the Natural Resources Defense Council's Ocean Initiative Benefit Hosted by Chanel on June 4, 2011, in Malibu.

And that's why I believe Melissa's journey to explore the evolution of style in LA, *City of Style*, truly is a celebration of Los Angeles fashion for what it is—unique. There is an eclectic flavor to this city, with women who embody many aspects of those who inspire them—from rockers to free-spirited bohemians to the modern, chic movie stars we all try to emulate (Gwen Stefani, in particular, is one style star that kills it in my eyes). In LA you never have to wear one head-to-toe look or monochromatic color. And that breeds a set of stylish inhabitants who aren't afraid to mix a Balenciaga jacket with a vintage, label-less sheath to make the look all their own and have a little fun.

LA gets a bad rap for its jeans and T-shirt culture. But, as Melissa explains, there's history and meaning behind the casualness. You'll never find girls in any other city who can pull off such a laid-back look while still remaining graceful. They own it, and that's what makes great style anyway.

Amber Valletta, SANTA MONICA
MODEL/ACTRESS

constraints of their corsets, personal style really did start in LA. And the basic fashion movements that started here can now be seen on billboards, television sets, and runways all over the globe.

Los Angeles is so relaxed that it sometimes feels uncomfortable to push boundaries when it comes to our fashion. But, luckily, you don't have to. Here, the sweet lace bra you wear peeking out from under your T-shirt is as important as the killer heels you'd wear running around in New York. A pair of perfectly fitting jeans is the equivalent to a structured day dress in Paris. LA has style. It's just very much its own.

Introduction

Upon moving from New York to Los Angeles in 2004, I thought I confidently had LA-style figured out as being one of two things: tight and short or beachy and casual. And while some of my expectations were met, the variations on style that started to emerge and become wholly apparent to me were striking and actually a bit awe-inspiring.

From subcultures to golden eras, I began to piece together my observations about several looks that not only felt organic to LA and its residents but also affect the way people all over the world put themselves together. A rare confluence of elements contribute to the LA lifestyle and to the kinds of looks that arise from living in a major city with ideal weather, a glamorous designer retail scene, and a celebrity and entertainment culture that doesn't just exist here: it was born here.

I set out to capture what I saw every day. Between running around designer showrooms downtown to lunch in Beverly Hills and after-work drinks in Venice, the people I encountered brought a vibrant and eclectic quality to what they wore. But an "LA look" isn't something that can be easily pinned down, and that's part of what makes it interesting, unpredictable, and fun.

LA-style is really like looking through one of those kaleidoscopes you had as a kid: glistening solid colors that when twisted and spun morphed into something more complex and more beautiful. It is colorful, eclectic, and often puzzling—and at its core, rich and inspiring.

The free-spirited energy, colorful sprawl of the city, and glorious sunny weather all undoubtedly inform the unique way LA denizens put clothing and accessories together.

And though LA has become synonymous with several mass-market trends, because of the casual nature of the ubiquitous daily uniform (think jeans, a T-shirt, and boots) there really is no cookie-cutter format, no formula or template to which people adhere. There's just a strong sense of individuality and creative self-expression that makes the city's style so appealing.

LA-style is ever changing and moving in a direction not solely dictated by what's happening on the runway. It blends the past with current trends and a lifestyle determined by the varied landscape, golden light, and sense of freedom.

In fact, freedom is the word that kept popping up throughout the research, interviews, and shared stories while writing this book. Whether people are rockers, hippies, or skaters, they describe their style as free. They are unencumbered in their clothing and look. Regardless if that means leather pants and boots or a floor-length dress made from old curtains, they feel free to move, make music, and flourish in their little piece of Los Angeles.

But while the past provides a rich history on which modern-day–style is built, a snapshot of the present is just as captivating.

By profiling stylish women and a handful of men, I got a glimpse of not only their personal looks and motivations, but also of the tapestry that comprises various inspirations coming out of LA. Each portrait offers a sense of discovery and a lesson in creativity and personal style. Subjects cite old film stars, friends, modern-day celebrities, mothers, and grandmothers when they talk about what drives their look. Their styles are nuanced and full of interesting details. No single person is a literal representation of the style under which they are categorized, but rather each manages to incorporate a unifying spirit into his or her appearance.

Walking into the homes and closets of people all over Los Angeles was not only the most informative and intimate way to get to know them but also to start piecing together the variety of styles that comprise this city. The subjects range from glamorous to supercasual, but they get dressed and live with a certain ease and insouciance that feels right for LA, whether that's been absorbed over time or something innate that has now found a place to thrive.

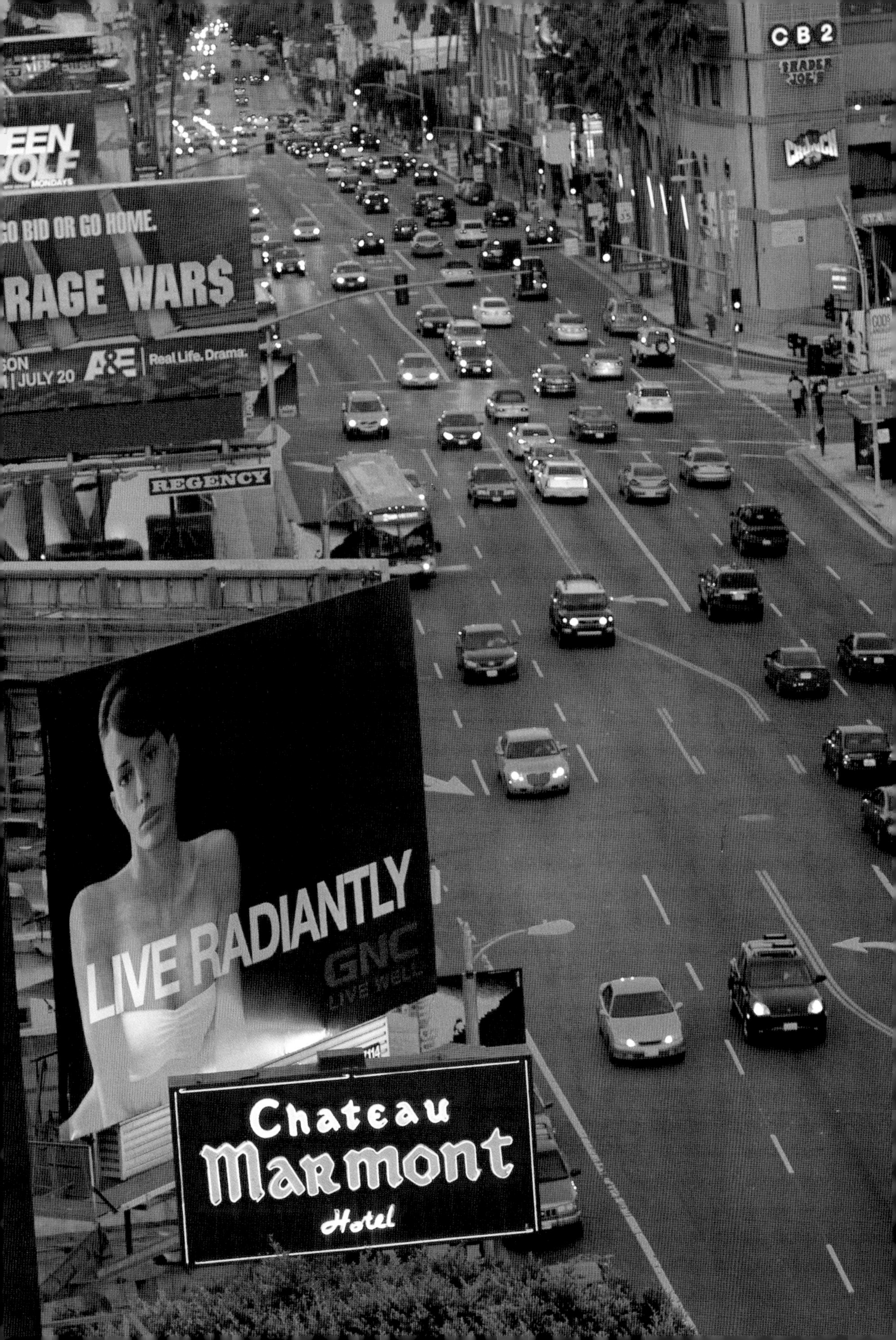
CB2
EEN
OLF
MONDAYS
O BID OR GO HOME.
RAGE WAR$
JULY 20
A&E
Real Life. Drama.
REGENCY
LIVE RADIANTLY
GNC
LIVE WELL
Chateau
Marmont
Hotel

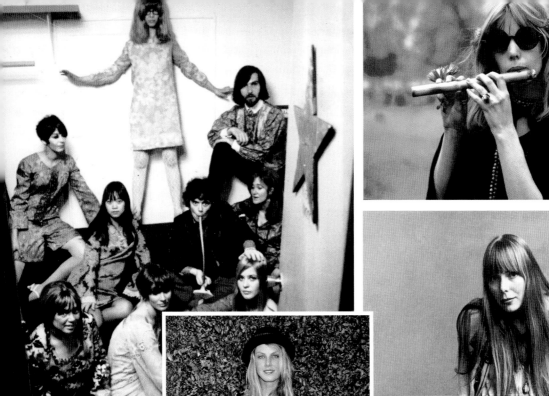

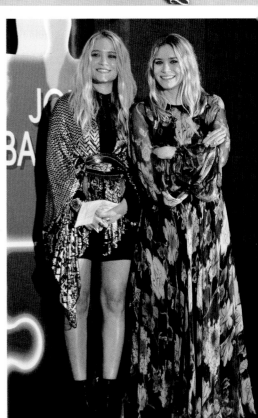

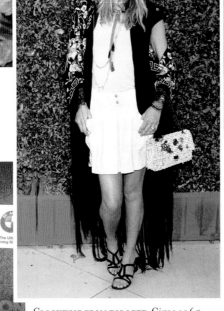

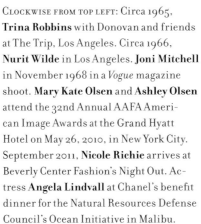

CLOCKWISE FROM TOP LEFT: Circa 1965, **Trina Robbins** with Donovan and friends at The Trip, Los Angeles. Circa 1966, **Nurit Wilde** in Los Angeles. **Joni Mitchell** in November 1968 in a *Vogue* magazine shoot. **Mary Kate Olsen** and **Ashley Olsen** attend the 32nd Annual AAFA American Image Awards at the Grand Hyatt Hotel on May 26, 2010, in New York City. September 2011, **Nicole Richie** arrives at Beverly Center Fashion's Night Out. Actress **Angela Lindvall** at Chanel's benefit dinner for the Natural Resources Defense Council's Ocean Initiative in Malibu.

romantic bohemians

I always think of the line Mama Cass sang, "... all the young girls are coming to the canyon." Those days you hitched your way up and it was perfectly safe. Talk about Camelot.

—TRINA ROBBINS

I f there's one style most commonly associated with LA, it's undoubtedly bohemian or "boho." The eclectic mix of vintage and denim works here like nowhere else, not only because of the casual, laid-back nature that permeates the city but also because of the hippie and musician counterculture that existed in the canyon neighborhoods during the 1960s. It can be seen today as a more literal interpretation of the romantic bohemians who dwelled in Laurel Canyon and frequented the love-ins in Griffith Park, or in updated details like fringe hanging off a slouchy suede bag and flare-leg, form-hugging jeans.

We're not talking overtly earthy tree hugger here. Even though the look is steeped in the free-spirited culture of the 60s and still embodies a more open-minded and laid-back attitude, LA girls have perfected a way of wearing the style (think stacks of string bracelets and the deliberate part down the center of their windblown hair) to include fashion-forward elements that are both free-flowing and sophisticated at the same time— ultimately a unique blend of contemporary fashion and a nod to the city's colorful canyon scene.

The wide-eyed musicians and artists who flocked to the

Laurel Canyon neighborhood in the mid-1960s marked the beginning of a movement that would inspire legendary songs and define a vibrant time in LA culture. The clothes they wore and the easy, unfussy nature of how they wore them also formed a template for the look as it is today. There is still the mix of DIY elements, long, loose shapes and rich embroidery on clothing and accessories that reflect the optimism of the 60s—a decade of change and new beginnings that's had a West Coast hub in the Canyon as well as in the nearby Sunset Strip that is still peppered with popular music venues.

There was a strong sense at that time that they had found the place where their music and ideas about art, politics, and culture could thrive among like-minded individuals in the enclave of Laurel Canyon, which provided a creative respite from the noise of the city.

The idealism of the 60s doesn't resonate as loudly in today's reality—but maybe that's why we're so unwilling to shake its style hallmarks, especially in LA, where driving through the Laurel Canyon neighborhood immediately conjures the ghosts of the musicians and artists who made an indelible mark on local style and culture. And certainly the carefree spirit associated with the boho look works just as well in the golden light and rambling sprawl of current-day LA.

The burgeoning boho aesthetic of 1960s LA also introduced the idea of more individual style, which drew a stark contrast to the band uniforms, prim petticoats, and pulled-together ensembles of the 1950s and early 60s. And, of course, it marked the emergence of some of music's most legendary and stylish figures—from Joni Mitchell to Frank Zappa.

The look of the LA scene at the time was partly built on the style of bands like the Rolling Stones—who broke through the mold of wearing band uniforms, like the Beatles before them—and began to dress in individual, not to mention relatively flamboyant, ensembles that couldn't help but garner the attention of and inspire anyone who saw them. The ears and budding urges of teenagers everywhere were suddenly piqued. And they took their sartorial cues not only from the Stones but also from local artists, including the Byrds, Buffalo Springfield, and Jim Morrison, embracing the sense of rebellion and adventure associated with the look, sound, and attitude of these musicians.

That idea of "doing your own thing" emerged around the same time, and suddenly young people's reality was more colorful and the prospect of self-expression was exciting and limitless. Much like LA itself, the era overflowed with optimism and endless possibility. In essence, both the scene and the music of Laurel Canyon worked to unite the energy of the city, the politics of the time, and the eclectic artists who were prolific and influential.

The standout details that were emblematic of this fresh and outrageous way of life came in the form of brocade, ruffled and romantic poet shirts, and nehru collars on tunic-style tops for men, and mini-length skirts and dresses (along with ankle-grazing maxi-length dresses) for women.

Bell-bottom silhouettes were also de rigueur for both men and women, as were sandals and made-to-measure moccasins. People began to look different and embraced their newfound freedom and various forms of expression, whether that meant a new sound in music, more introspective lyrics, or bold flourishes on clothing that echoed the individualism, artistic license, and electric energy people felt during the decade and in the city.

This sense of individuality was seen in both the men and women who embraced the open-minded lifestyle rooted in Laurel Canyon. Singer Joni Mitchell famously wrote some of her best-known songs while living in the neighborhood, along with other notable musicians of the time like Cass Elliott, Jim Morrison, and David Crosby. Her song "Ladies of the Canyon" painted a vivid picture of several of the women living and creating in the Canyon. One of those was Trina Robbins, who's specifically mentioned in the lyrics as sewing and designing clothes, which she did during the mid-60s in LA for the likes of Mitchell, Crosby, and Elliott.

Robbins was always a clotheshorse, so when she moved into Laurel Canyon in 1960, she bought an old sewing machine and locked herself in a room where she started sewing dresses, shirts, and bell-bottoms for her friends.

"Word got around that I made great clothes," says Robbins, who crafted velvet bell-bottoms, paisley shirts, and brocade jackets for people to wear every day or while performing onstage. The black minidress she made for Mitchell was something the iconic singer would layer over her bell-bottom pants, a silhouette not unlike the tunic length tops women today pair with skinny jeans or leggings.

Fashion—even among successful musicians and artists—was much more egalitarian than it is in our current designer-label-obsessed climate, with women swapping clothes freely, buying secondhand, and reworking fabric from unexpected sources.

Case in point: Robbins fashioned a dreamy-looking long dress with bell sleeves and a tiered skirt out of old lace curtains for Enid Karl, former girlfriend

corey lynn calter

I like how girls put things together here; there is a casual hipness to their style that seems very natural. For me, California has always been indicative of the Joni Mitchell/Laurel Canyon/Malibu, laid-back bohemian lifestyle. Fashion here is about really stylish girls who have fun with clothes in a very free and playful way.

of folk singer Donovan and mother to musician Donovan Leitch and actress Ione Skye. And she created a pair of red velvet hip-hugging bell-bottoms for Jim Morrison's girlfriend, Pamela Courson. The ladies also favored miniskirts, maxidresses (also known as "granny dresses"), halter tops, and elaborate embroidered bell-bottom pants.

Nobody settled for just roughed-up jeans. They punched up the look with satin or silk bell-bottoms, or outfits made out of brocade or velvet. "You *dressed* for acid," says Robbins. "You would wear a floaty something or beads . . . You dressed for whatever activity you were engaging in. The girls in LA wore shorter skirts than the ones in New York, but I suppose LA has always been more outrageous."

Tie-dye and paisley were the two most ubiquitous prints. There was a local spot for handmade tie-dye called the Farm, according to journalist Harvey Kubernik, which was a commune nestled off Lankershim Boulevard at the base of the north side of the Hollywood Hills. It was there that a woman who fittingly went by the name of Tie Dye Annie, made tie-dyed pieces for various musicians.

The DIY mentality and hunger for custom-made clothing were a direct reflection of the time—as independent, individual, and eclectic as possible. Perhaps that's why most clothing was made by hand out of natural fabrics that could only be found at specific shops like Bob Steinberg's Fabric Emporium, a rambling and musician-friendly store on Melrose Avenue.

Janis Joplin, Jimi Hendrix, and Mick Jagger frequented the Fabric Emporium if not for the vast array of psychedelic patterns and robust selection of paisley, then for the laid-back vibe that was conducive to hanging out. Steinberg claims that getting stoned every morning, opening the shop at 1:00 PM, and not closing until 9:00 PM was a way of life at the time, and the hours and atmosphere lent to the store's location becoming a bustling hub for creative types immersed in 60s counterculture.

Steinberg had a "no polyester" policy, and carried only natural fibers and what he boasts was the largest selection of paisley prints around. Paisley was easily one of the defining prints of the time and it could be seen not just on Jimi Hendrix's shirts, but covering the furniture sitting in hippie pads or festooning the seats in their vans.

In addition to stocking an impressive quantity of paisley prints, Steinberg claims that his store was the first to start selling tie-dye fabric over the counter. He charged the hippies who walked in wearing tie-dye shirts with the task of dying the white fabric he gave them, and then bringing it back in so he could sell the hand-dyed cloth. He also merchandised the store to be as much a visual experience as it was a retail outlet, setting up each room by where the fabric or print was from. One room was filled with exotic, earth-toned prints from Africa while the next had a dizzying color wheel's array of bright and metallic fabrics from India. "I sold inspiration. I sold art by the yard. It was a temple of material reality," says Steinberg. He recites his fabric store's catch phrase from the 1960s and it's not hard to imagine what the scene was like—acid-bright colors, bold paisley prints, handmade hippie tie-dye, and all. "I'm a fabric man, faster than a bolt of speeding paisley, crazier than a quilt. Young and old, hip and straight, black and white, they all unite at the Fabric Emporium!"

While the boho look is long, loose, and flowy, the clothing was ultimately about feeling free and uninhibited about what you were wearing. Items like miniskirts and dresses that didn't require a bra or any underpinnings started surfacing and again mirrored the free attitude and feeling of exuberance buzzing at the time.

A shop owner named Charles Lange stocked his store, Belinda Boutique, with items that went minimal on the fabric and heavy on the flash and glamour. The items drew a stark contrast to the earth-mother hippie look, with miniskirts, slinky fabrics, and dresses suitable to be worn without a bra. In fact, *Vogue* magazine credited Lange's boutique as having brought the miniskirt to the West Coast, and the abbreviated bottoms were what his customers—who included Grace Slick, Sharon Tate, and Tina Turner—flocked to the store to find.

Belinda Boutique relished shedding 1950s conservative clothing and gave women the option to wear pieces that were not only less stuffy, but that also required few or no undergarments. It was quite a drastic change from the cumbersome corsets and underpinnings that shaped women just a few years earlier, but according to Lange, the expression of freedom and the feeling of liberation that arose from this new style of clothing reflected the political climate and escalating music scene throughout the country. It was a place where many young people put their foot down against war and traditional notions of patriotism. And their fight was expressed not only through protests or music, but also in the 180-degree shift in what they wore compared to the previous decade.

The notion of individual expression resonated even louder with the musicians and performers of the day, and to ensure getting the most unique and eye-catching clothing, they went to local designers like Ola Hudson, who created ensembles for people like Cher, Linda Ronstadt, John Lennon, David Bowie, and Ringo Starr. The LA native and mother of Saul Hudson (a.k.a. Slash of Guns N' Roses) set up a few stores in the West Hollywood area where clients could pop by to have her design something personal and stage ready.

Hudson's artistic prowess and connection to the entertainment industry would influence her son, who shares her carefree and eclectic approach to dressing.

"She was always very artistic and a really fluid illustrator," he says. "She really understood the human form and how to drape clothes on it. She was really fun and free spirited."

Boho-style remains one of the most romanticized and emulated forces in fashion, popping up in the collections of Gucci, Stella McCartney, Anna Sui, and Roberto Cavalli in recent seasons.

"A lot of people want to embody the spirit of LA-style—cool, easy, and usually with a hint of boho," says designer Jill

Stuart, who has tapped the look for several of her collections. She adds that no one ever wants to look like they tried too hard or put too much thought into their outfit, and LA girls especially have mastered the ease of getting dressed.

Designer Corey Lynn Calter agrees, admiring not only how the bohemian look is worn in LA, but consistently referencing the easy shapes and colorful palette for her spring and resort collections. Whether it's gauzy dresses with floral embroidery or a light and airy colorfully printed top, the free-flowing fluidity of the clothing worn in LA from the 60s to today remains parallel not only in look, but also attitude.

"The way people wore clothes was really a reflection of who they were," says celebrity stylist Meritt Elliott, who, along with Emily Current, designs the denim label Current/Elliott. "Until the 60s it was taboo to look outrageous. It was the first time in history people were able to wear clothing that reflected their personal style."

"People lived together, made music together, and clothing became a hodgepodge of your personality on your body," adds Elliott.

Current and Elliott not only tap the era for their denim line—creating distressed cutoff jean shorts, high-waist bell-bottoms, and worn-looking chambray shirts and denim jackets—they also conjure up the boho feeling for their celebrity-styling clients, who include Emma Roberts and Mandy Moore. Denim not only has a relaxed aesthetic, but starting in the 1960s

it became a symbol of eschewing the sartorial formality expected during the 1950s and early 60s.

The duo deliberately dress their clients, both actors and musicians, in a free-spirited boho look when the person is promoting an album or doing something related to music, because they claim that it automatically gives the artist a feeling of creative armor and a style more grounded in the exuberance of the 60s Laurel Canyon scene.

"The look is not overtly sexy," says Calter about the way boho-style is worn today. "Girls look effortless and there's something inherently cool about that. Plus, there's a vibe you give off when you wear these boho-inspired pieces. It changes you somehow."

Clothing played a role in the transformation of a generation during the 1960s. Fashion is a direct reflection of what is happening socially and politically and in this decade it was glaringly obvious. Silhouettes went from pulled together and uniform to loose and airy. Political statements were made through patches with slogans or sayings, unkempt hair, and bright color.

The feeling still visibly resonates throughout the city today, whether driving through the labyrinth of narrow streets in the Canyon or seeing an LA girl dressed in flared jeans, a loose and light tank top, and, of course, piles of pristine gold bangles mingling with threadbare bracelets that look like she could have made them herself.

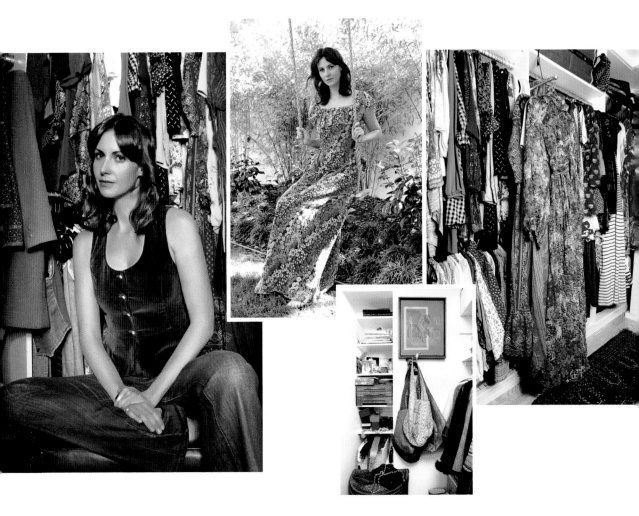

Name: LIZ CAREY   **Hometown: TOLEDO, OHIO**   **Occupation: comedienne**

How would you describe your style?
I'm torn between hippies and 1970s disco ladies. I love a long and flowy number or a peasant blouse, but I do also love a good jumpsuit.

What are your go-to pieces?
My go-to pieces are always vintage. Right now that's a vintage wool plaid cape from Pendleton and a yellow dress from the Rose Bowl Flea Market that I swear is

Ossie Clark with the label missing. It was only nine dollars and I'm still congratulating myself.

Who are your favorite designers?
Ossie Clark, Chanel, Jane Mayle, and the dollar bin outside of Hidden Treasures in Topanga Canyon.

What is your signature scent?
Fracas mixed with patchouli oil.

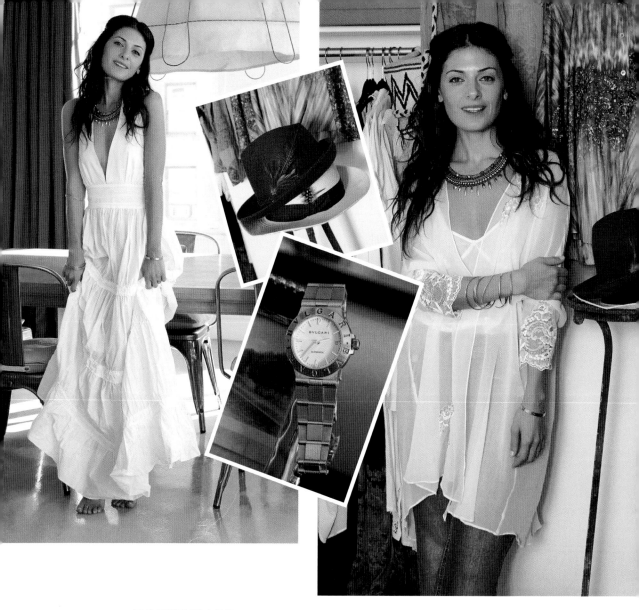

Name: RONIT NABI   Hometown: LOS Angeles, CA   Occupation: STYLIST

How would you describe your style?
Romantic, simple, understated.

Who are your style icons?
Jane Birkin's French tomboy style. And Brigitte Bardot's sexy hairstyles are addictive.

What are your go-to pieces and favorite items in your closet?
My go-to pieces are high-waist jeans, white T-shirts, vintage slip dresses, and long, flowy dresses. My favorite item is my gold Bulgari watch given to me by my husband as a wedding gift.

What is the last thing you bought?
A snake-shaped ring and an Isabel Marant tunic.

Who are your favorite designers?
Phoebe Philo, Dries Van Noten, Isabel Marant, Stella McCartney.

What is your signature hairstyle?
Wavy, unkempt hair, parted down the middle.

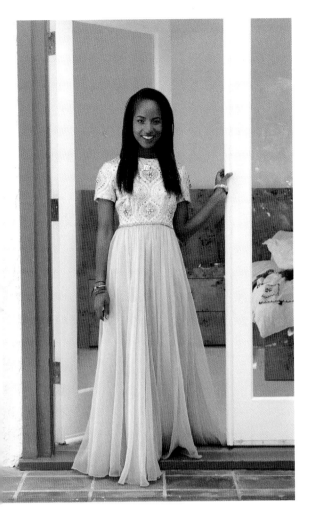

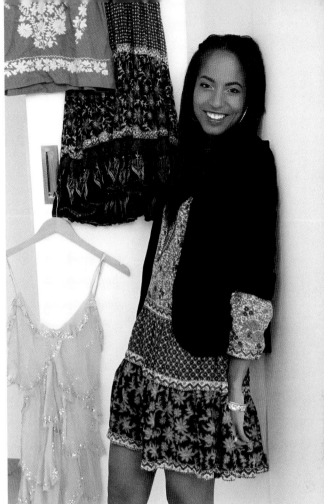

Name: **WELLS BUTLER**   Hometown: FAIRFIELD, IA
Occupation: FASHION DESIGNER

How would you describe your style?
Whimsical and eclectic. I mix and match girly with androgynous, bohemian with classic prep.

What are the go-to pieces in your closet?
If I could only wear one style of clothing for the rest of my life it would be vintage dresses. I wear dresses with everything: blazers, hoodies, sandals, and heels.

What is the last thing you bought?
A 3.1 Phillip Lim sweater with tuxedo tails. I love clothing that has unexpected whimsical details.

Who are your favorite designers?
Erin Fetherston, 3.1 Phillip Lim, Vanessa Bruno, and Matthew Williamson.

Name your signature scent, hairstyle, hair color, or other things you feel distinguish your style.
Jo Malone's Nectarine Blossom and Honey perfume and Fresh's Citron de Vigne. I always channel the 70s with my hair. It's either down and parted in the middle with waves or braided. And I can't leave the house without my layers of bracelets. I feel naked without them.

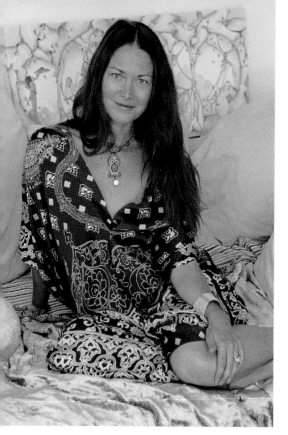

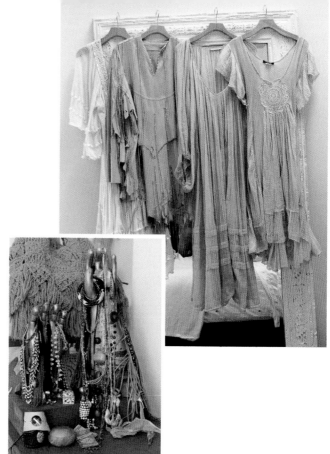

Name: CARRIE JARDINE   Hometown: CaLGary, ALBerTa   Occupation: ArTIST

How would you describe your style?

I dress how I feel at the moment. I will wear anything from my long billowing Pucci or gauzy Calypso beach cover-up belted as a dress with a nude mesh Cali Dreaming bikini underneath, to a crisp, white Ralph Lauren button-down and my Dolce & Gabbana skintight white pencil skirt. I like to mix it up with an eclectic blend of various styles.

Who inspires how you dress?

I'm inspired by the aesthetic of North American Native cultures, art nouveau, the 70s, and European fashion in the late 1700s to early 1800s.

What are your favorite items in your closet?

My favorite items are my Martin Margiela cognac leather and Lucite heels. They make everything special. And my majestic, hand-embroidered necklace by Dori Csengeri is absolute perfection!

What would you consider a signature aspect of your style?

Color, I rarely wear black.

What is the last thing you bought?

Four beautiful golden rings, one for each finger, by Gabriela Artigas and a gorgeous long white and peacock print caftan by Camilla.

Who are your favorite designers?

I love Matthew Williamson. He's amazing.

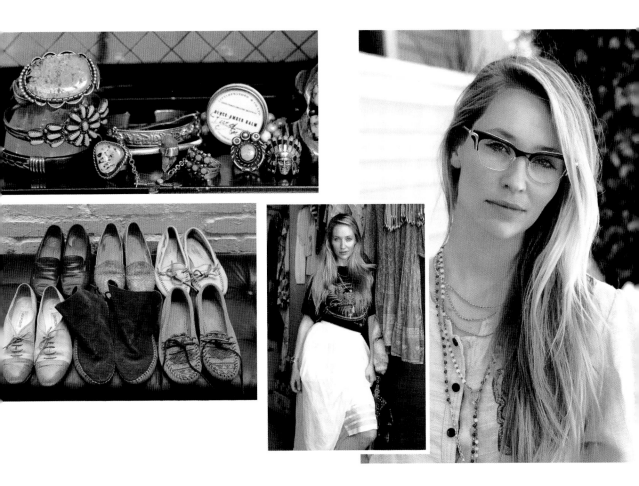

Name: BAELYN ELSPETH   Hometown: EAST LOS ANGELES, CA
Occupation: CO-OWNER OF A VINTAGE BOUTIQUE

How would you describe your style?
Some days I want to be a flower child and run around barefoot with a muumuu on. Other days I feel preppy and want to wear loafers, silk tops, and cashmere sweaters. But ultimately, the ability to feel free in clothing is extremely important. I don't want to be boxed in by any particular style or trend.

What are the go-to pieces in your closet?
I have a black cotton jumper that I live in, and a few muumuus that I would die without. And I love the vintage Native-American jewelry my mom gets me in New Mexico.

Who are your favorite designers?
I don't really have one. I like different things at different times and I don't think any one person gets it exactly right every time with every piece. That being said I find myself inspired by pieces from Ralph Lauren, Helmut Lang, and Jenni Kayne. Everything the designers at Heyoka Leather do is hot.

Name your signature scent and hairstyle.
Black Amber Balm from Little Feather, Kiehl's Musk, and No. 17 from Sebastian Signs. My hair is always blond, long, and natural.

Do you have any clothing or accessory items you wear daily or almost daily?
Everyone knows me for my glasses.

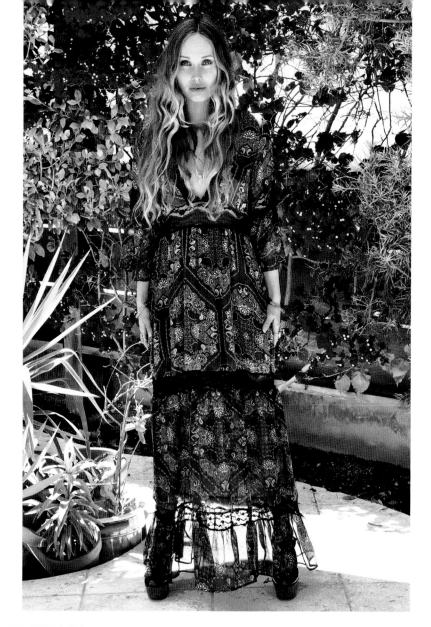

Name: **EMILY CADENHEAD**   **Hometown:** MALIBU AND PALM SPRINGS, CA
Occupation: DESIGNER

How would you describe your style?
Bohemian meets American gothic.

Who are your style icons?
My style icons are my grandmothers, who both had a wonderful sense of fashion and personal style.

What is the last thing you bought?
A pair of 1970s raw crystal earrings that look very *Mists of Avalon*.

Who are your favorite designers?
Kansai Yamamoto, Tao Kurihara, and Issey Miyake.

Name your signature hairstyle, hair color, or other things you feel distinguish your style.
My hair is very long and natural. I rarely blow-dry or style it. Platform sandals, lots of rings, bright colors, and I never leave the house without a hat!

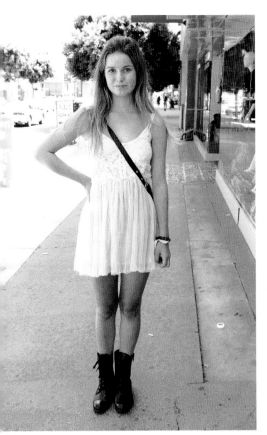

Name: ERIN KINCAID
Hometown: NEWPORT BEACH, CA
Occupation: STUDENT

How would you describe your style?
My style reflects my free spirit. It changes daily but every outfit has a touch of bohemian to it.

Who are your style icons?
My style icon is Isabel Lucas. Most of her clothes come from flea markets, thrift stores, and vintage shops and she manages to make them look both feminine and chic.

What would you consider a signature aspect of your style?
A touch of bohemian always does the trick and a wrist full of different bracelets.

Who are your favorite designers?
Marc Jacobs and Alexander Wang.

Name: MIWA SAKAMOTO
Hometown: SANTA MONICA, CA
Occupation: STUDENT/MODEL

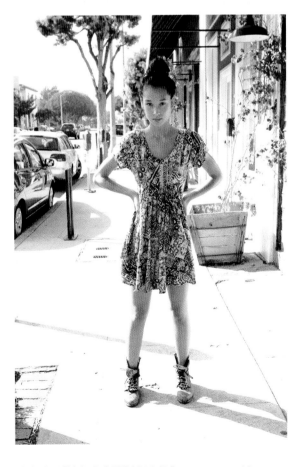

How would you describe your style?
My style is really a million things and whatever catches my eye. Usually that's Native/hippie/minimal and maybe a little grunge. I love the sun-kissed California ease with a little edge.

What are the go-to pieces in your closet?
Vintage Levi's and clogs.

What is the last thing you bought?
Some supersick books by Becca Moon at A. Kinney Court.

Who are your favorite designers?
Alexander Wang, Rick Owens, Dries Van Noten, Raquel Allegra.

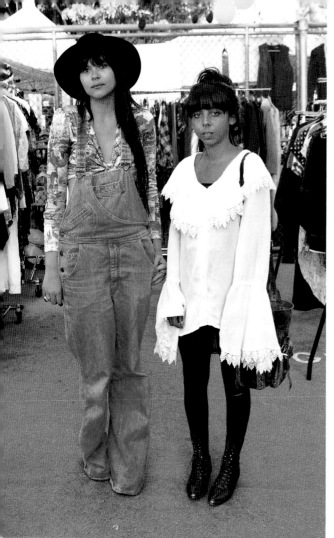

Name: **ENAIA GREBER**
(On left, in overalls)
Hometown: LOS ANGELES, CA
Occupation: Jewelry Designer

How would you describe your style?

My style ranges from whimsical 70s to dark western gypsy, with lots of rich decadent colors and plenty of black. And you'll almost never see me without a hat on!

Do you have any style icons or count any films as inspiration?

My style icons are 70s Alice Cooper and those 60s–70s Biba girls. I usually count more on musical inspiration than films, so I'd have to say dark Stevie Nicks meets Neil Young and Black Sabbath.

What are your go-to pieces and favorite items in your closet?

My black, wide-brim velvet hat, and my favorite dress, which is a very simple, low-cut, black floor-length dress from the 70s. It is mysterious and complemented by tarnished belts and silver jewelry.

What would you consider a signature aspect of your style?

A signature aspect of my style would have to be mixing dark and whimsical elements from different times and worlds to create something that's all my own.

What is the last thing you bought?

I just bought a bunch of tiny antique silver western belt buckles, which I'll use to make bootstraps and hatbands.

Who are your favorite designers?

I love vintage Norma Kamali from the 70s, Alexander McQueen, and Gucci (especially the Fall 2008 collection. It blows my mind!).

What are your beauty habits? Do you have a signature scent?

Sugar body scrub, face toner, bangs, cat-eye makeup, and pink lollipop lip balm. My signature scent on a sweet day is Versace Bright Crystal and for wild nights I go with Dior Pure Poison.

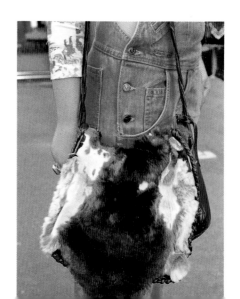

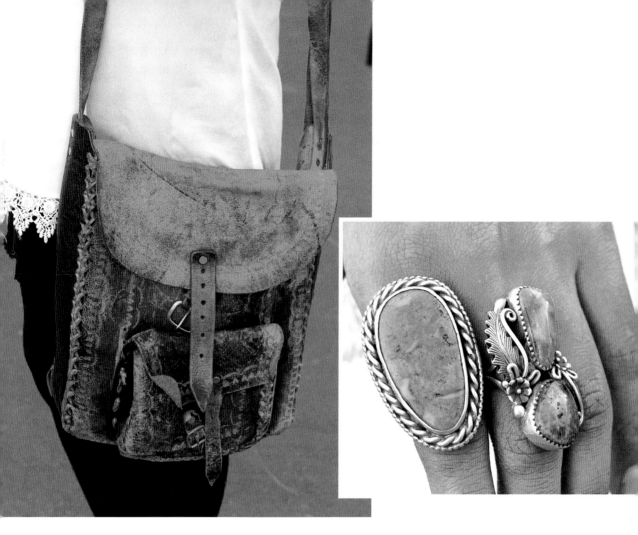

Name: **JOHNIQUE SHACKELFORD**
(Oppostie, right, in white dress)
Hometown: VENICE BEACH, CA
Occupation: CLOTHING and JEWELRY DESIGNER

How would you describe your style?
I would describe my style as 70s bohemian punk, gypsy-rock goddess.

Who are your style icons?
Anita Pallenberg was BAD-ASS in the 70s. I'm pretty influenced by her, as well as Keith Richards. I adore the movie *Performance*, starring Anita Pallenberg and Mick Jagger.

What are the go-to pieces in your closet?
Turquoise jewelry, wide-brim hats, and vintage platform shoes.

What is the last thing you bought?
The last thing I bought was a pair of vintage silver boot tips and heel guards.

Who are your favorite designers?
My favorite designers are Barbara Hulanicki (Biba), Jessica McClintock (Gunne Sax), Pendleton, and Acne.

What are your beauty habits? Do you have a signature scent?
Trimmed bangs, a clean face, exfoliating pads, and liquid eyeliner are a must! My signature scent is Viva la Juicy by Juicy Couture.

HIDDEN TREASURES

154 S. Topanga Canyon Blvd.
Topanga, CA 90290
(310) 455-2998

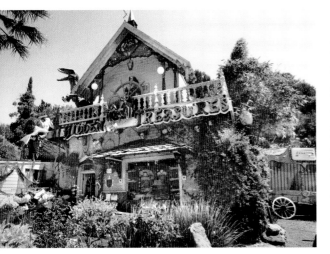

Housed in a whimsical setting that's part hippie hideaway, part fairy-tale fantasy, Hidden Treasures is tucked away atop Topanga Canyon and is a destination for people who want a trippy shopping experience and affordable, interesting vintage clothing.

Owner Darrell Hazen started selling vintage wares on the side of the road in Topanga Canyon in the 1970s and eventually set up this brick-and-mortar shop. Focusing on pieces from the 1920s through the 1970s, Hidden Treasures is a multiroom store with a layout that meanders and winds around, adding to the quaint experience and element of surprise. New merchandise is added every two weeks to keep the place brimming with men's, women's, and a small selection of children's clothing and accessories.

Despite the broad selection, the store's best-selling items seem to fit the location and look of where they're housed. Long, flowing muumuus, light and gauzy cotton dresses, bohemian-style dresses, and leather jackets from the 1960s and 70s are hot items for shoppers who make the trek up to Topanga or pass through on their way to the beach.

Body-skimming dresses from the 1930s as well as fur coats are a big hit with models like Kate Moss, who has referenced Hidden Treasures as one of her favorite shopping spots when interviewed about her style.

Prices remain reasonable—$145 for a 1920s-era beaded dress. And there's an even less expensive option for real bargain hunters at the $1.75 box that sits in front of the store, where crafty and creative shoppers can find items to alter or wear as is. Talk about a hidden treasure.

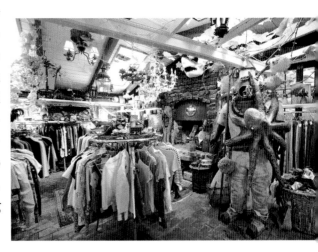

ROSE BOWL FLEA MARKET

1001 Rose Bowl Drive
Pasadena, CA 91103
(626) 577-3100

Built in 1921, the Rose Bowl stadium has become a cultural crossroads not only for music performances, sports, and arts and crafts fairs, but since 1967 the expansive grounds surrounding the arena have also been transformed into the Rose Bowl Flea Market, attracting hipsters, hoarders, tourists, and teenagers all looking to peruse the over twenty-five hundred vendors selling quirky collectibles, antique jewelry, old magazines, and just about everything a vintage clothing connoisseur could ever want.

Flea market vendors clearly follow trends and stock items that attract fashion-hungry shoppers. If the 1920s are in, you're bound to find more drop-waist dresses and long strands of beads and pearls; if the 80s are de rigueur, fluorescent details, black pointy-toed boots, and bright leather crossbody bags might make a strong appearance. But the mainstay look at the flea market is 1960s and 70s boho, which can be found in the dozens of stalls featuring old leather boots, turquoise jewelry, endless tables of distressed leather belts, and, of course, the booths packed with vibrant, embroidered Mexican dresses, flowy and colorful caftans, and paisley-printed broomstick skirts.

Designers from all over the world as well as local creative types looking for inspiration head to the flea market for pieces to reference or a spark from the past to inform their current-day collections.

Not only is the location an exciting and relatively inexpensive source for vintage clothing and furniture, there are plenty of men and women walking the grounds who serve as stylish muses for anyone who wants to see how vintage wares and trendy pieces come together in Southern California.

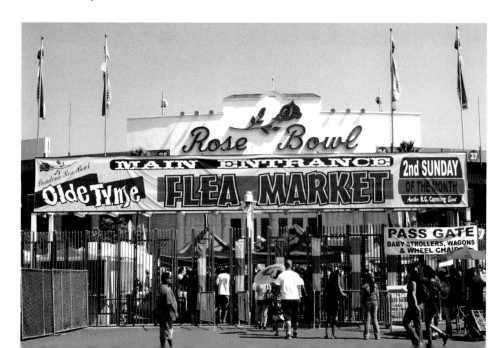

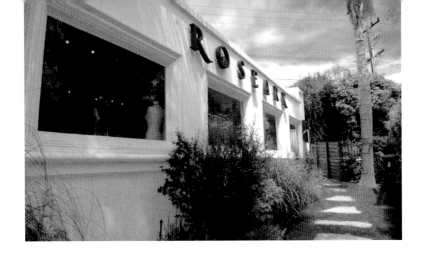

ROSEARK

1111 N. Crescent Heights Blvd.
Los Angeles, CA 90046
(323) 822-3600

Rarely concealed by woolly scarves or gloves, jewelry is on display year-round in LA, where the temperate weather is a big reason so many stylish girls pile on stacks of bangles both chunky and skinny and mix their string bracelets with diamond-smattered cuffs. From the dainty to the weighty and sculptural, jewelry is a major part of a Southern California girl's style, and the store Roseark carries a vast array of feminine and bohemian pieces to pair with long, flowy gowns or everyday denim cutoffs and gauzy tops.

Owner and designer Kathy Rose opened Roseark in 2007. The 5,000 square foot boutique nestled in West Hollywood houses not only jewelry, but moccasins, home objects, and art as well (Rose also opened a second location in Santa Monica in 2010). She carries about two hundred different lines of jewelry in the store and due to Rose's extremely selective eye, you're not likely to see the same things that saturate mass-market department stores. She also likes to support smaller designers, many of them local tal-

ent who find exposure through the constant daily rotation of stylists and celebrities who walk through Roseark's doors.

"You can be any size and jewelry is great on everyone," says Rose, who also designs her eponymous line of nature-inspired jewelry. Think sexy rose gold snake bracelets that wrap around the forearm or earthy arrowhead pendants set in gold and diamonds. "I notice that my clients don't buy things just to buy them. They add on and it becomes their art pieces. You can really build your own collection of heirlooms."

Rose displays these potential heirlooms in various rooms throughout the space. There are areas for tribal jewelry, art deco–inspired pieces, and estate pieces as well. Rose gold is a big passion for Rose, who not only carries a lot of it, but also makes many of her own designs in the pink-tinged metal. She says that LA customers gravitate toward earthy designs like arrowheads, eagles, snakes, and feathers. "It's like they're adding more talismans to their collection."

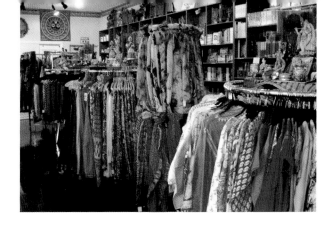

GOVINDA'S

3764 Watseka Ave.
Los Angeles, CA 90034
(310) 204-3263

On a side street in Culver City, situated right next to the Hare Krishna temple, sits the most unassuming of shops called Govinda's International Imports. The non-profit store has been aboveGovinda's vegetarian restaurant there since 1986, under the direction of buyer and manager Tadit Beca, who stocks the store with an almost dizzying array of clothing, shoes, scarves, jewelry, bags, and quilts all handmade in India.

The traditional and fashion forward together in the form of bright floral patterns hand embroidered at the neckline with neon pink thread or neutral ikat-print tops that feel like a designer's resort collection come right off the runway—and fortunately for a small fraction of the high-end price. "Women who can afford anything come in and mix high with low," says Beca. In addition to buying for the store, she commissions artisans in various regions of India to create prints made with hand-carved wood blocks and dyed with all natural pigments like turmeric, pomegranate, and indigo. She has also been bringing in one-of-a-kind brightly colored patchwork bags

made from pieces of antique wall hangings, which have inspired contemporary designers to create look-alike versions but with a much heftier price tag than the boldly hued and delicately embellished bags that hang in Govinda's.

"Color is an opulence that transcends price," says Beca. "It's cheerful and happy and doesn't have to be expensive." Color also comes in the form of the hand-painted whisper-light cashmere scarves, sets of gold bangles with splashes of red and green, and silver jewelry sporting vivid natural stones. Most of the jewelry is made by a process in which the craftsperson takes tree sap, pours the resin into a mold, and wraps the piece in a sheet of silver. This keeps the jewelry light and less expensive, with earrings selling for $8–$10.

Rounding out the abundant selection of handcrafted clothing and accessories, Beca stocks all-natural bath and beauty products, including soap, lotion, aromatherapy oils, and floral-scented waters.

"I always saw the shop as a great way to integrate with the community and provide an oasis to anyone who comes in."

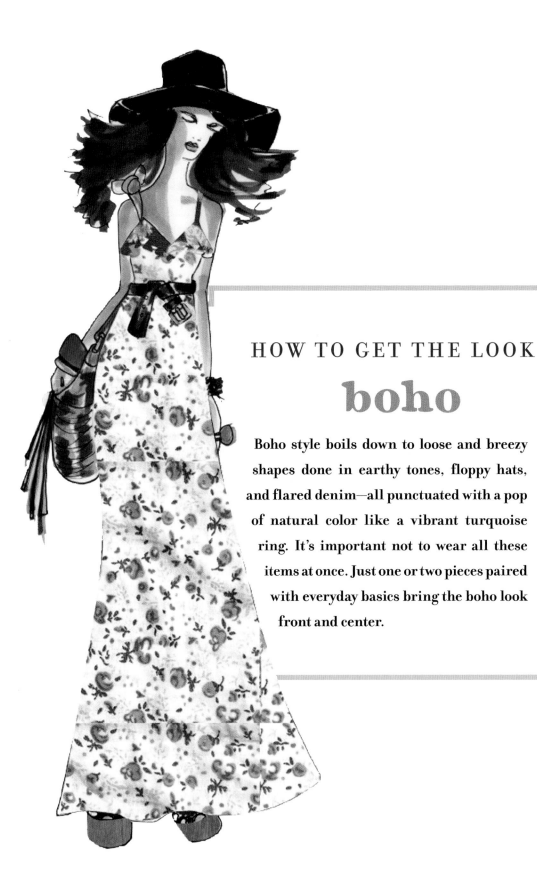

HOW TO GET THE LOOK

boho

Boho style boils down to loose and breezy shapes done in earthy tones, floppy hats, and flared denim—all punctuated with a pop of natural color like a vibrant turquoise ring. It's important not to wear all these items at once. Just one or two pieces paired with everyday basics bring the boho look front and center.

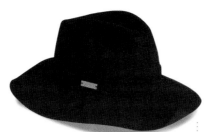

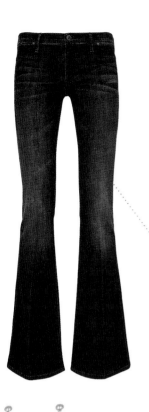

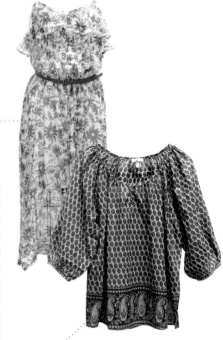

Flare leg or bell-bottom-style jeans are a casual boho staple.

A floppy, wide-brim hat tops off the relaxed look.

Throw on a long floral dress that has an earthy yet feminine vibe. Wear it long, loose, and flowy, or cinch it with a worn-in leather belt.

An airy ethnic-print top pairs well with jeans or cutoff shorts.

Colorful pops of jewelry punctuate muted earth tones.

Brown suede moccasins are a comfortable and genuine boho basic.

Ankle strap wedges are a dressier option that still have a boho vibe.

Tangles of leather and beaded bracelets look haphazard but chic.

Hammered gold bangles add a bit of polish while still looking down-to-earth.

A suede hobo bag with fringe is the quintessential boho accessory.

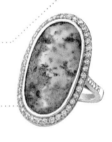

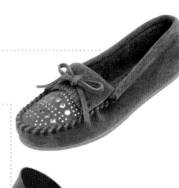

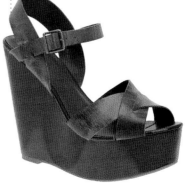

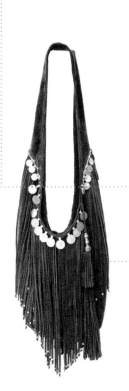

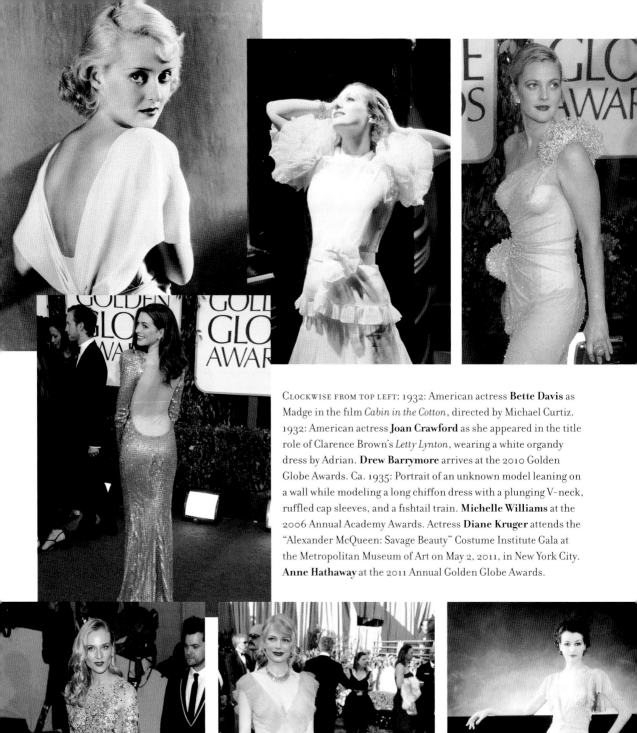

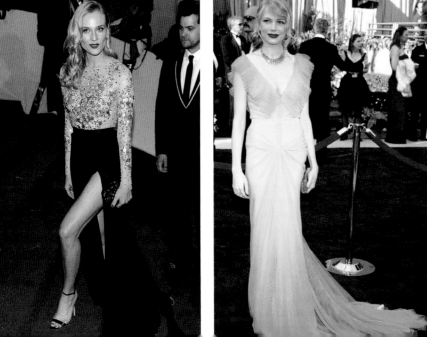

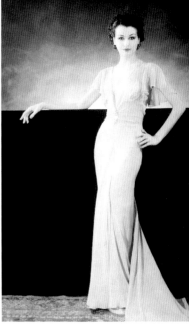

Clockwise from top left: 1932: American actress **Bette Davis** as Madge in the film *Cabin in the Cotton*, directed by Michael Curtiz. 1932: American actress **Joan Crawford** as she appeared in the title role of Clarence Brown's *Letty Lynton*, wearing a white organdy dress by Adrian. **Drew Barrymore** arrives at the 2010 Golden Globe Awards. Ca. 1935: Portrait of an unknown model leaning on a wall while modeling a long chiffon dress with a plunging V-neck, ruffled cap sleeves, and a fishtail train. **Michelle Williams** at the 2006 Annual Academy Awards. Actress **Diane Kruger** attends the "Alexander McQueen: Savage Beauty" Costume Institute Gala at the Metropolitan Museum of Art on May 2, 2011, in New York City. **Anne Hathaway** at the 2011 Annual Golden Globe Awards.

glamour

Old Hollywood is about celebrating a woman's body, not challenging it.
—GEORGINA CHAPMAN

The look of Old Hollywood is a recurring theme from high-end designers to contemporary collections. Whether it's an obvious nod to the era or a subtle detail on a modern-day dress, the glamour of the 1930s and 40s in Hollywood is seen and felt just about everywhere.

The glamorous, ultrafeminine style of Old Hollywood has been mined countless times on runways, on the street, and in popular culture. Just cruise down Hollywood Boulevard's souvenir row—where the image of Marilyn Monroe in her white halter dress with the provocatively flowing skirt adorns mugs, T-shirts, and posters—to witness its unwavering influence.

Why? Our appetite for celebrity and fantasy is ultimately insatiable, and few eras have offered more unabashed glamour than the golden age of cinema in Hollywood.

Jean Harlow's platinum blond finger waves, Joan Crawford's strong padded shoulders, and the nipped waistline of an elegant Audrey Hepburn are among the more recognizable details that remain inextricably linked to the look and mystique of the era.

Silver screen icons Joan Crawford, Lauren Bacall, Jean Harlow, Marilyn Monroe, Grace Kelly, and Audrey Hepburn possessed ravishing good looks and were dressed by the best studio costumers of the day. Wardrobe wizards Gilbert Adrian, Jean

Louis, Edith Head, and William Travilla all worked within Hollywood's studio system, carefully crafting memorable clothing as well as personas: the public's perception of the industry's biggest stars.

Hollywood's studio system—from 1929 to the early 1950s, when the creation of television changed the dynamic of movies—is often referred to as the industry's golden age. The biggest studios, such as MGM, Paramount, and Warner Bros., developed talent and dictated not only the movies they starred in and the parts they played, but also their hairstyles and overall looks—all to project a specific image to a public that became fascinated with the glamour and allure of the final product.

"There is a mystery [to Old Hollywood] and that is why it's potent," says Kevin Jones, museum curator at the Fashion Institute of Design & Merchandising in LA, about why the glamour of Hollywood's golden age continues to endure. "The studios controlled everything. The movie stars were told what to do, what to wear, and how to wear it." He adds that the in-house costume designers created clothing to fit the specific look and reputation of the studio. MGM was known for glamour. Warner Bros. was about noir. Stars under contract with the studios were expected to carry out the look from the screen to their private lives so the magic behind each studio and its stars remained a mystery.

The magic of those movies and its stars was particularly appealing during the late 1920s and early 30s as an escape from the grim reality of the Great Depression. Movie stars were elevated to icons and the clothing they wore became something to aspire to. Costume designers were not only the behind-the-scenes forces for how each actress was presented to the public, but they also enhanced each one of their on-screen characters to fit studios' expectations and fulfill audiences' hunger for glamour and fantasy.

A few of the most notable costume designers to contribute legendary looks to Old Hollywood set the bar for glamour as we know it today.

Perhaps one of the most heralded and prolific costume designers of Hollywood's golden age was Adrian. Born Adrian Adolph Greenberg, he sometimes went by Gilbert Adrian—though his on-screen credit always read "Gowns by Adrian." The designer joined MGM in 1928. It was at MGM where Adrian made an indelible mark not only in film, but also in the way on-screen looks affected fashion. He is often credited with creating the strong-shouldered style of Crawford and setting in motion the silhouette as a trend for both the actress and millions of women during the mid-1930s.

Adrian also famously worked with Judy Garland, creating the iconic ruby red slippers and blue-and-white gingham dress for Garland's character in *The Wizard of Oz*. In 1941, Adrian left MGM to open his own store in Los Angeles selling his gowns and glamorous creations to the public.

Irene Lentz was Adrian's successor at MGM, signing on as head costume designer in 1942. Lentz had experience dressing starlets prior to landing at MGM. As the head of Bullocks Wilshire Ladies Custom Salon, she began working with actresses like Myrna

Loy and Claudette Colbert and created delicate and glamorous evening gowns that gained her a stellar reputation for designing pieces that were both ultrafeminine and flattering.

Lentz's abilities went beyond just making beautiful gowns. In the nearly two hundred films designed over her eight years at MGM, Lentz made costumes that spanned from soft and pretty to strong and confident to altogether racy and exotic like Lana Turner's turban and hot pants look from *The Postman Always Rings Twice*.

Travis Banton began at Paramount Studios in 1924—an ideal time to arrive—as their roster was filled with some of the biggest stars of the day, including Marlene Dietrich, Carole Lombard, and Claudette Colbert. He designed the costumes for films such as *Shanghai Express*, *The Dressmaker from Paris*, and *A Farewell to Arms*, and he was known for understated elegance and exceptional use of the best fabrics. He also created a few iconic looks that endure today. Banton's menswear-inspired costumes for Dietrich in her films *Morocco* and *The Scarlet Empress* kick-started what became a signature look for the star.

> ## joe zee
>
> *LA isn't secondary to what's happening in style and design anymore. We live in a fabric of pop culture now and can't deny that LA is important. LA influences what we do day-to-day. Award shows aren't about awards anymore. People can't remember who won an award but can probably tell you who looked best.*

Today that menswear-inspired look continues to be a recurring trend on runways as well as a foundation of style for many women who love the ease and insouciance of androgynous dressing. Trousers, boxy blazers with strong shoulders, and flat lace-up oxfords are all direct descendants from golden era Hollywood fashion of the 1930s and 40s and the style of stars like Dietrich.

With her signature round spectacles, blunt bangs, and cropped hairdo, Edith Head is nearly as recognizable as the boldface names she dressed during her forty-year career as a costume designer.

Head created costumes for some of history's most heavily referenced movies when it comes to fashion. Head's costumes for movies such as *Roman Holiday*, *To Catch a Thief*, *Sabrina*, and *Funny Face* not only enhanced the beauty (and performances) of the actresses who starred in them, but also helped build a body of work that designers, stylists, and celebrities still reference for inspiration today.

The look of Old Hollywood is still ubiquitous and the most obvious place to see its unabashed glamour on parade is on LA's red carpets, specifically the entertainment industry's biggest celebrations like the Academy Awards and the Golden Globes, which impact style trends as profoundly as any runway show. In recent years the most breathtaking moments in fashion have happened on Hollywood's red carpet—with actresses clad in classic gowns from designers like Dior, Marchesa, Reem Acra, and Armani Privé that strongly echo styles from Hollywood's golden age.

"Nostalgia is a very strong chord to pluck," says vintage retailer and fashion expert Doris Raymond, citing a number of old-school-style hallmarks that still survive. For example, lingerie-style dresses associated with the bias-cut silk gowns of Jean Harlow convey everything from demure ingenue to sultry vixen, a classic chignon implies grandeur and old money, and finger waves allude to a sultry look.

"There is safety in being inspired by sure things," says luxury-brand consultant and vintage retailer Cameron Silver. "And you really can't go wrong with an Audrey Hepburn LBD or a slip dress like ones Jean Harlow wore. Those looks will always be desirable."

Glamour is all about the details, whether that means understated, delicate fabrics like lace or more overt, shiny touches like sequins and beading. These key details used during the golden era of Hollywood are still relevant today—glittery accents and sleek silhouettes that seem never to go out of style.

Bugle beads and beading in general lent sparkle and a sense of opulence and importance to a movie character back in the day. Beading is not only lustrous and attractive in photographs, it demonstrates consummate craftsmanship—as hours of labor are involved in creating a single beaded dress.

Lace is undoubtedly the most efficient way to convey femininity and, sometimes, innocence. It can be dramatic if done in a dark color like black, which was the most commonly used hue in the films of Old Hollywood. But wrought in white or a light pastel, it looks almost ethereal—as evidenced by the lilac lace Elie Saab gown Mila Kunis wore to the 2011 Oscars.

Bias-cut gowns were a signature of the 1930s, and Jean Harlow is nearly as famous for her bias-cut frocks as she is for her platinum blond locks. Bias-cut gowns drape gently, subtly accentuate curves, and tend to be more flattering than solid pieces of fabric for the skirt portion of a gown.

As in the films of the 1930s and 40s, a plunging back will forever convey sexiness and confidence. While the gowns of Old Hollywood may not have been as revealing as contemporary dresses are, an open back projects just as sultry an image.

A signature element of Joan Crawford's style, the broad-shouldered look, influenced everyday fashion in the 1930s and 40s. This eventually led to the power shoulder of the 1980s and early 90s, but on the red carpet we still see this style dramatically played out with interesting flourishes on the shoulder, which convey a sexy boldness and the ability to take a fashion risk.

When awards season descends on LA in the very early spring, the glamorous feeling of Old Hollywood increases considerably. The electricity that pulses through the city is palpable and for some the speculation over which dresses the top stars will wear is just as titillating as the suspense over who will end up winning an award. Starlets are ushered around town from fitting to fitting, their stylists plucking jewels, dresses, and accessories to complete a sartorial puzzle steeped in age-old glamour.

Although today's definition of celebrity has been slightly diluted—the studio system of Old Hollywood created an aura of mystery and inscrutability around its stars that couldn't possibly survive today's 24/7 paparazzi culture—our expectation of high glamour and fantasy remain. People still want the fantasy despite knowing what goes on behind the scenes.

We still watch awards-show red carpets with the same fervor we always have. We're addicted to the gorgeous parades of gowns, jewel-encrusted clutches, and bevy of borrowed baubles that drip from wrists, necks, and ears despite the advent of social media, the Internet, and reality television that have exposed the nuts and bolts of how the glamour all comes together. The curtain has been lifted and the mystique diminished, but nothing has changed about our fascination with red carpet fashion.

And is that so bad? The absence of mystery isn't necessarily a negative thing (we even know which facialists, gifting suites, and salons the celebs patronize to prep themselves for a big night), but it certainly exposes the machinery of the Hollywood glamour apparatus.

We know each celebrity stylist's name, and perhaps even how many gowns their star client tried on before deciding on the winner. Still, the barrage of information doesn't really affect the glistening, opulent outcome of major red carpet events—or how jazzed we are to finally see the glamorous pieces coalesce.

"There is still stardust in our eyes," says Jones. "The difference is that the making of a star used to be more authentic. Now it's not as much, yet the desire for it is still 100 percent."

Designers today understand this modern desire for glamour, and they create their collections around the fantasy churned out by Hollywood.

"Old Hollywood is so influential for all of us," says Georgina Chapman, codesigner of red carpet heavyweight label Marchesa. "It represents a glamour and beauty you never step away from as a designer, because it's always about making a woman look as beautiful as possible. Old Hollywood glamour is about celebrating a woman's body, not about challenging it."

Chapman and her design partner, Keren Craig, are known for making some of the dreamiest, most glamorous gowns today. The styles range from Grecian goddess–

inspired to long, frothy, and highly embellished. They celebrate the opulence of Hollywood and the red carpet while applying just enough restraint for each design to remain elegant, tasteful, and attractive on the stars who wear the dresses and to the audience watching them at home.

LA-based special occasion designer Kevan Hall echoes Chapman's sentiment. "I love to reference Old Hollywood," says Hall, whose Stage Door collection several seasons ago was inspired by Garbo, Shearer, Dietrich, and even Adrian.

Full of bias-cut gowns, heavy, luxurious fabrics, and fur and feather flourishes, the collection continues to reference Old Hollywood's pulled together and polished aesthetic. Regardless of whether a star was casual or dressy, there was still a consistent sense of style in place.

Reem Acra, whose glam gowns are a red carpet staple, admits that she thinks about Old Hollywood every time she designs. "Even at five years old, I always looked at [images of Old Hollywood stars] and wanted to imitate the look. The reference is always going to be in my designs, but always with a twist—a modernized version."

Taylor Swift, Olivia Wilde, and Nicole Richie have all worn Acra's gowns to award shows, showcasing the designer's sensibility for ethereal yet polished dresses.

Celebrity stylist and television fashion personality George Kotsiopoulos adds that today's glamour lies in looking classic, effortless, and polished all at once, but that nothing trumps personality. For example, "Angelina Jolie wears her clothes; her clothes don't wear her," he says. "You can look back on photos of her years from now and they'll be timeless."

In our modern-day world of fast-paced fashion, Old Hollywood stands out as a constant source of inspiration. The timeless, classic nature of the stars who wore the looks continues to represent an ideal of glamour, sensuality, and mystery.

While glamour is a given on the red carpet, the style can also be seen every day on LA streets. Glamorous elements punctuate even the most casual outfits in LA. It is apparent in the status bags, fur-trimmed outerwear, and fully made-up faces of women strolling down Rodeo Drive and the adjacent streets in the heart of Beverly Hills. It's a living, breathing part of each day in the city where glamour was born and perfected.

MONIQUE LHUILLIER

My red-carpet dresses are very much a reflection of modern-day Hollywood Glamour. Women in LA tend to dress more casual and relaxed during the day, but at night they now how to get dressed and make a statement!

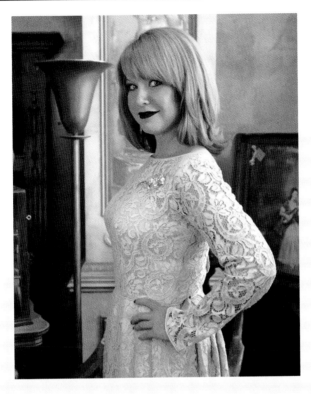

Name: **SHANA HONEYMAN**   Hometown: LOS ANGELES, CA
Occupation: PUBLIC RELATIONS DIRECTOR

How would you describe your style?
Valley of the Dolls **meets** *Steel Magnolias*.
I don't wear jeans or flats and am always armed with a powder brush and lipstick. I love to have a sense of humor with my wardrobe, and I don't mind that my best friend once mistook a senior citizen in a pink Chanel suit for me from afar, which was the ultimate form of flattery!

Who are your style icons?
My style icons are Lana Turner in *Imitation of Life*, Catherine Deneuve in *Umbrellas of Cherbourg*, Dolly Parton, Carol Channing, Phyllis Nefler, the Lawrence Welk girls, and of course, my mother.

What are your favorite pieces in your closet?
The items I covet the most in my closet are my collection of Vivienne Westwood hand-bags, a pair of Sonia Rykiel rhinestone-encrusted heels, a black Rami Kashou pencil skirt that instantly transforms my shape into an hourglass, my collection of whimsical Corey Lynn Calter dresses, and my mother's violet Christian Dior wedding dress she married my father in.

Who are your favorite designers?
Sonia Rykiel, Vivienne Westwood, Zandra Rhodes, Corey Lynn Calter, Rachel Comey.

What is a signature element that you feel helps distinguish your style?
My hair is definitely the trait that distinguishes my style. I have had every version of a retro hairstyle from Doris Day to Tammy Wynette.

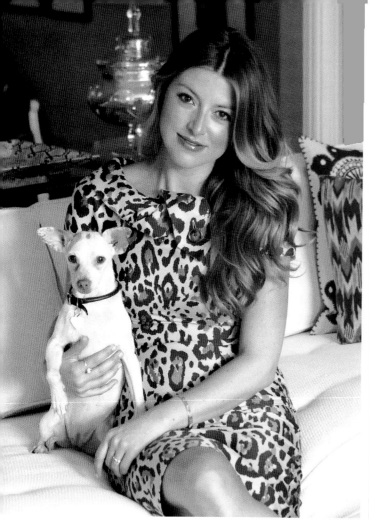
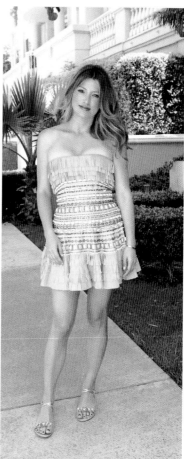

Name: **SARA RIFF**   Hometown: Laguna Beach, CA
Occupation: Fashion Publicist

How would you describe your style?
Classic with a bit of an edge, feminine and
a little glam. I gravitate toward body-
conscious silhouettes and stay far away
from anything too flowy or shapeless.

Who are your style icons?
I love Natalia Vodianova. She is so stunning that everything looks perfect on her.
Georgia May Jagger is supersexy and pulls
off over-the-top glam without looking like
she is trying too hard, which I think is the
ultimate achievement. I'm drawn toward
superconfident women who can carry off
all different kinds of looks with tremen-

dous spirit and confidence—women from
Bianca Jagger to Diane Keaton to Diane
Kruger to Diane von Furstenberg (I have
a thing for Dianes!).

**What are your favorite items in your
closet?**
My Balenciaga leather jacket was a
splurge and I have never looked back.
Anita Ko panther earrings. My feathered Marchesa cocktail dress and Yves
Salomon cropped fur coat, which looks
amazing with everything from black
tie to jeans. My amazing collection of
Jimmy Choo shoes, Jenni Kayne snake-

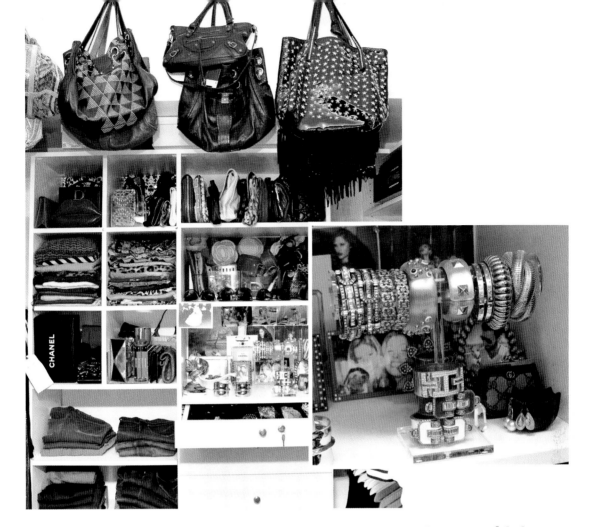

skin motorcycle jacket, Vince jeans, Lulu Guinness red lips clutch, Louis Vuitton leopard scarf . . . somebody stop me.

And what would you consider a signature aspect of your style?

Fashion should be fun and I think my style tends to be playful. I love mixing unexpected accessories to dress up casual looks and I'm not above "theme" dressing. Leopard print is my favorite color.

What is the last thing you bought?

An Hermès Medor watch in black with gold spikes, which I had to track down on eBay. Various wild shades of Chanel nail polish. And I just received the most fabulous chrysoprase Irene Neuwirth earrings as a gift that adds a colorful *pow* to any look.

And what is your must-have piece of clothing right now?

A fabulous black lace trench coat, it looks amazing with anything or nothing at all.

Name your signature scent, hairstyle, hair color, or other things you feel distinguish your style.

I combine fragrances to create my own custom scent and mix it up like a little chemist depending on my mood. My hair is a golden caramel color, which I tend to wear long with a loose curl. I don't know that I have ever seen myself without lip gloss. That's definitely my signature, although I love a red lip.

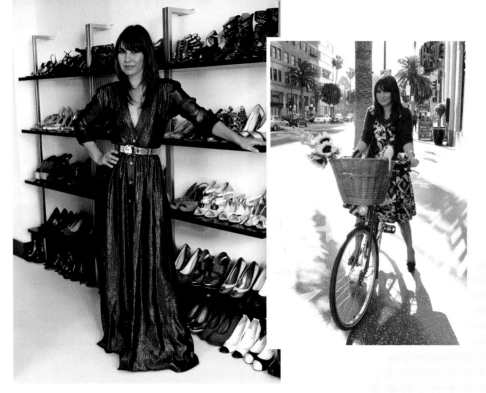

Name: NICOLE CHAVEZ   **Hometown:** LOS ANGELES, CA
Occupation: CELEBRITY STYLIST

How would you describe your style?
My style is eclectic, ladylike, and tailored. I love color and bold animal prints like zebra and ikat. I love ethnic prints for that world traveler vibe.

What are your go-to pieces and/or your favorite item in your closet?
A leopard print three-quarter sleeve YSL dress; it's such a go-to and I love it. And every single Etro piece I have, for the heavy prints.

What is the last thing you bought? And what is your must-have piece of clothing right now?
I just bought a red-and-white-striped skirt and blue-and-white monkey shirt from Prada. I wish I could wear it every single day. It's so quirky and witty and silly and bright and I love that. I wear the striped skirt a lot with a white T-shirt or gray sweatshirt or even mix it up with more stripes. I love mixing patterns.

Who are your favorite designers?
I love Prada, especially the accessories, Jenni Kayne, Oscar de la Renta, Chanel, and Duro Olowu for the prints. Valentino—it's so feminine, light, and pretty.

Name your signature scent and hairstyle.
My signature scent is Chanel Coromandel and my bangs are kind of a signature.

Do you have any clothing or accessory items you wear daily or almost daily? If yes, what are they and why are they meaningful to you?
A gold coin bracelet that belonged to my grandmother that I'm obsessed with, and a black diamond band with a garnet in the center from my sister. I live with my Louis Vuitton rolling suitcase; I'm never without it. I pack my life in that bag and take it from my house to my office every day. It's a carry-on size and it has a section for my iPad and my computer, and room for one outfit, makeup, and workout clothes.

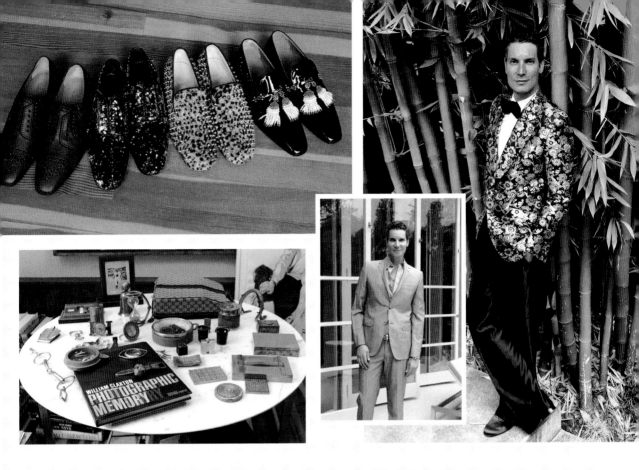

Name: **CAMERON SILVER**   Hometown: LOS ANGELES, CA
Occupation: RETAIL AND LUXURY BRAND CONSULTANT

How would you describe your style?
 Eclectic iconic.

Who or what inspires how you dress? Do you have any style icons or count any films as inspiration?
 Style icons include Baron de Rede, Cary Grant, and Dirk Bogarde. Inspiring films are *The Eyes of Laura Mars*, *North by Northwest*, and *Diva*.

What are your go-to pieces and/or your favorite item in your closet? And what would you consider a signature aspect of your style?
 A tux jacket, tux shirts, black skinny Levi's, Gucci loafers, man bling, great man bag. My style is very day to evening and a little tongue-in-cheek, nothing basic, nothing boring, and not a lot of black.

What is the last thing you bought?
 A Rod Keenan hat.

Who are your favorite designers and your go-to places to shop?
 Alexander McQueen, Bottega Veneta, Louis Vuitton, Rick Owens, Phillip Lim, Acne, Jean Paul Gaultier, Brunello Cucinelli, Jil Sander, Costume National. My favorite stores include Opening Ceremony in Los Angeles, Isetan in Tokyo, Barneys in New York, and flea markets in Paris.

What are your grooming habits? Do you have a signature scent?
 Erno Laszlo for skin, Frederic Fekkai for hair, Dr. Perricone for vitamins, and my scent is Frederic Malle Geranium Pour Monsieur.

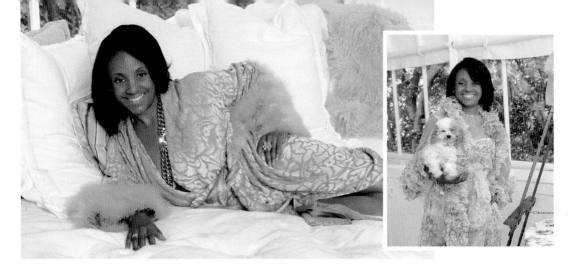

Name: RONA STEVENSON **Hometown:** CHICAGO, IL
Occupation: CURATOR OF COUTURE AND DESIGNER VINTAGE CLOTHING,
ACCESSORIES, AND ANTIQUES

How would you describe your style?
A mix of 1920s, 1930s, 1970s, and 1980s glamour, mixed with classic preppy lady chic. I love everything from seersucker to chiffon, sequins, and fur.

Who or what inspires how you dress?
My daily wardrobe inspiration comes from my feelings, the location, temperature, and the classic movie I watched the night before.

Who are your style icons?
My mother, Frieda Lee. She's beyond chic and has fun with fashion. I grew up in Chicago with her fur closet, shoe closet, *L'Officiel* and *Vogue* magazines. Other style icons include Diana Ross, Nancy Reagan, Bianca Jagger, Daphne Guinness, and Kate Moss.

What are your go-to pieces in your closet?
A beige cashmere cable-knit sweater that I wear all year. It's like my baby blanket and I take it everywhere. Chanel handbags; they are a classic staple that works with any of my looks whether it's seersucker or sequins. I always wear a heel with the exception of proper tennis whites and yachting attire.

And what would you consider a signature aspect of your style?
The mix of vintage and new and the blend of classic lady chic with ultraglamorous pieces, a lot of silk chiffon, Grecian dresses, caftans, dresses made a little sexier with a heel, cashmere, and fur—I need the balance. I'm a Libra.

What is the last thing you bought? What is your must-have piece of clothing right now?
The most amazing 1970s Chloé silk dress and new Chanel tan suede over-the-knee boots. They're thirty years apart, but both Karl Lagerfeld.

Who are your favorite designers?
Chanel/Karl Lagerfeld, vintage and new; Yves Saint Laurent, vintage Valentino, vintage Halston, vintage Ungaro, James Galanos, Geoffrey Beene, Stavropolus, and Arnold Scaasi.

Name your signature scent, hairstyle, hair color, or other things you feel distinguish your style.
My hairstyle depends on my mood and look of the day, but it's usually soft loose curls with slight feathering to channel Jaclyn Smith and Farrah Fawcett in *Charlie's Angels* **circa 1976.**

Name: MARC CIRENO   Hometown: LOS ANGELES, CA
Occupation: FINANCE

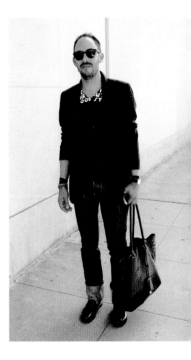

How would you describe your style?
Modern, minimal to Donald Judd–like proportions.

Do you have any style icons?
My style icons are Steven Meisel, Helmut Lang, and Yves Saint Laurent.

What are your go-to pieces and/or your favorite item in your closet?
My go-to pieces are a black tuxedo and white French cuff shirts. My favorite item is an Hermès "Bad Boy" belt.

What is the last thing you bought?
Lanvin trousers.

Who are your favorite designers?
Martin Margiela, Rick Owens, Azzedine Alaïa.

Do you have a signature scent?
Comme des Garçons Parfum.

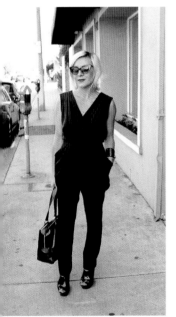

Name: ERI HOXHA   Hometown: LOS ANGELES, CA
VIA EUROPE   **Occupation:** STYLE CONSULTANT

How would you describe your style?
Confidence and good manners.

Do you have any style icons or count any films as inspiration?
Marchesa Casati for her individuality, and Audrey Hepburn, because she carried herself with such grace. Films are definitely an inspiration—Kar Wai Wong's *In the Mood for Love* and Claude Lelouch's *A Man and a Woman*, to name a few.

What are the go-to pieces in your closet?
Whenever I am in doubt, I wear a black dress—I have so many, so I always have an option depending on the occasion.

What would you consider a signature aspect of your style?
A signature aspect of my style is heels. I'm always in high heels—every day, everywhere.

What is the last thing you bought?
A vintage YSL blouse from the Rive Gauche Spring 1979 collection.

Who are your favorite designers?
Yves Saint Laurent, Valentino, and Raf Simons.

What are your grooming habits?
Skin care is very important to me. I use a lot of Chanel products. I always use toner for my face, and I do my own nails.

Do you have a signature scent?
It changes depending on the mood, so these days it is Violet Blonde by Tom Ford.

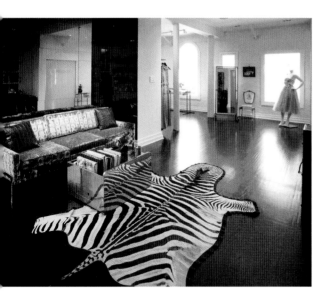

DECADES
8214½ Melrose Ave.
Los Angeles, CA 90046
(323) 655-0223

In 1997, when Cameron Silver opened the doors to his vintage vault on Melrose Avenue, grunge was all the rage and glamour seemed to be on hiatus in the fashion world. Silver became inspired to present vintage clothing in a modern format and bring a refined element to fashion when everything was just the antithesis.

The result of his vision has become one of the most influential shops and collections both for women who appreciate the history behind a classic piece and celebrities who don vintage gowns from Decades when gliding down the red carpet. Twenty-first-century fashion icons, including Jennifer Lopez, Victoria Beckham, and Gwyneth Paltrow have shopped at Decades. Silver has created several of the most memorable Hollywood-style moments.

Remember that canary-yellow Jean Desses gown Renée Zellweger wore to the 2001 Oscar awards? Or more recently, Kristin Davis in a creamy white vintage Balmain dress with a beaded bust and cap sleeves as well as a shimmering gold, halter-neck Norman Norell gown during the swirl of press calls and premieres for *Sex and the City 2*?

Silver has spent years acquiring his broad mix of twentieth-century pieces, and the hunt for amazing items is never finished. He is constantly buying items from women selling their designer wares, at auction or sometimes sight unseen—just going on his keen sense for a vintage gem. But to Silver, vintage does not mean retro. Every gown, bag, pair of shoes or earrings that sits in the selection at Decades has a feeling of modernity and carefully makes its way to its new owner with Silver's deft guidance.

"The fun for me is not knowing where a piece might end up," he says. "That's the game. I want to find it a home and make a good match between the garment and the wearer."

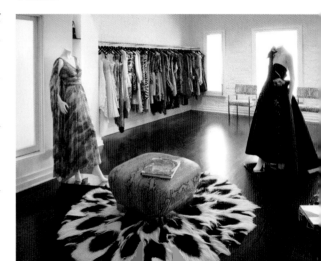

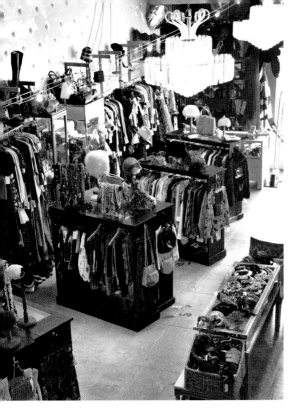

THE WAY WE WORE
334 S. La Brea Ave.
Los Angeles, CA 90036
(323) 937-0878

Her shop is filled to the rafters with 1970s Halston dresses, 1950s Dior and Galanos dresses, jewelry and belts from the 1940s, and *Dynasty*-style sequined cocktail numbers from the 1980s. Walk in on any given day and you're bound to see LA residents and fashion-savvy shoppers such as Rachel Bilson, Kelly Wearstler, and Mia Sara thumbing through the racks of clothes or sifting through baskets of scarves and belts. Raymond has also supplied some of the world's most important designers, such as Marc Jacobs, Anna Sui, John Galliano, and the late Alexander McQueen, with vintage items that serve as inspiration for their collections each season.

"I realized that clothing designers had a huge appetite for good inspirational pieces and I began to see more designers coming on a frequent basis," she says. Raymond took over the retail space next door to The Way We Wore and quickly filled the storefront with archival pieces that designers can peruse and buy for inspiration purposes.

To keep her store stocked with covetable vintage wares, Raymond spends about a quarter of the year on the road on buying trips all over the country. And though her journeys always prove fruitful, there is still the search for her "holy grail" of vintage finds. "I would love to find a Charles James ball gown," says Raymond. "I think I would stop breathing if I found one."

It started with a triangle-shaped carnelian ring purchased secondhand in Marin, California, over twenty years ago that sparked Doris Raymond, doyenne of LA vintage fashion, to start down a path of extensive collecting as well as learning the history and details behind most of the gems she scours on international buying trips. "Someone made a comment about Egyptian revival when seeing that carnelian ring," says Raymond. "I didn't know what he was talking about, so I went to the library to do research and that's when I fell in love with the art deco movement. That planted the seed for my curiosity for the 1920s, which expanded into fashion and accessories."

And the rest, as they say, is history. Raymond has been a serious collector of vintage clothing and accessories for twelve years and opened her store, The Way We Wore, on La Brea Avenue in midcity Los Angeles in May 2004.

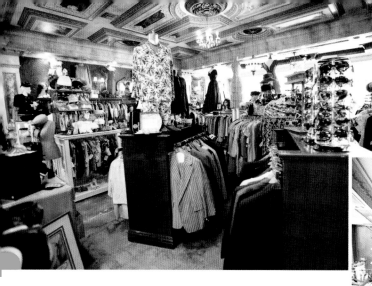

PLAYCLOTHES

3100 W. Magnolia Blvd.
Burbank, CA 91505
(818) 557-8447

Imagine a dress-up chest on steroids filled with poufy party dresses, marabou-lined slippers and robes, and houndstooth swing coats all in immaculate condition. That's essentially what Playclothes feels like—a packed-to-the-rafters treasure trove of vintage clothing, accessories, collectibles, and furniture in Burbank. The 4,000-square-foot space houses pieces from the 1930s through the 1980s all organized by color-coded tag denoting the decade.

Owner Wanda Soileau is an ex-dancer who has always had a passion for vintage clothing. After selling at flea markets in LA for several years, she eventually opened her own store, which has occupied several locations in the San Fernando Valley for the past seventeen years.

Now located on a quaint corner of Magnolia Blvd. in Burbank, the store is a haven for women who love to search through vintage gems primarily from the 1940s, a decade Soileau is infatuated with for its classic silhouettes and hourglass-shaped Joan Crawford–style suits.

In addition to 1940s suits and dresses, there are Charles Jourdan shoes, costume jewelry, a rack of 1960s pajamas, vintage furs, and furniture—including distressed patio furniture, gliders, and gold-and-glass end tables. The selling floor is packed with merchandise, which covers almost every surface, nook, and cranny.

In fact, Soileau works closely with a lot of studios and costume designers who buy items for the characters they dress for TV and film. Janie Bryant, costume designer for *Mad Men,* has been buying clothes for the Madison Avenue ad execs on the show since the first season and she continues to be a regular customer both professionally and personally.

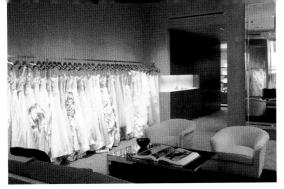
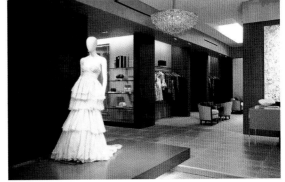

MONIQUE LHUILLIER
8485 Melrose Pl.
Los Angeles, CA 90069
(323) 655-1088

When it comes to the ultimate in beautiful bridal gowns and special occasion pieces, Monique Lhuillier is a go-to location for women and celebrities planning a dream wedding or gearing up for a glamorous event. The LA-based Lhuillier's creations have been worn by everyone from Carrie Underwood and Pink to Mila Kunis and Reese Witherspoon. Her flagship boutique in the quaint shopping area of Melrose Place houses both her frothy gowns and all the items that round out the elegant and ultra-glamorous lifestyle she projects.

Lhuillier's bridal line was founded in 1996, and her boutique sits in the posh Melrose Place locale, where it's wholly apparent how much her collection has expanded into a full luxury lifestyle brand. There are wedding gowns, ready-to-wear, handbags, and a tabletop line all available for purchase in the 4,200-square-foot store. The location originally housed an antiques shop that had been there for twenty-two years, and the corner locale still carries the charm and interest it did when antiques were sold there.

Lhuillier was inspired by her own home when planning and decorating the store—which has taupe, embossed-lizard wall wrappings, warm ash paneling, and soft-hued natural gray stone—and she aimed to make the store feel like an inviting residence. The gallery of the store features a central sculpted skylight and the salon has translucent wall panels. French and American vintage furniture from the 1940s, 60s, and 70s are in the space, as well as custom-made pieces, created especially for the boutique. Paul Evans, Edward Wormley, and Milo Baughman are some of the sculptors featured there.

Lhuillier's evening-wear collections, first introduced in 2002, take up a large portion of the store. Jessica Alba, Catherine Zeta Jones, Gwyneth Paltrow, and Scarlett Johansson are among the stars who have worn her gowns on the red carpet. Lhuillier's bridal gowns are displayed in a dedicated section of the store, where starry-eyed brides-to-be can peruse the selection and try on their dream dress.

A collection of small bags and clutches are available exclusively in Lhuillier's stores. Bags are made mostly with exotic skins such as snakeskin and ostrich. There is also fine china giftware that features colors and details that correspond with the signature sashes of her wedding gowns.

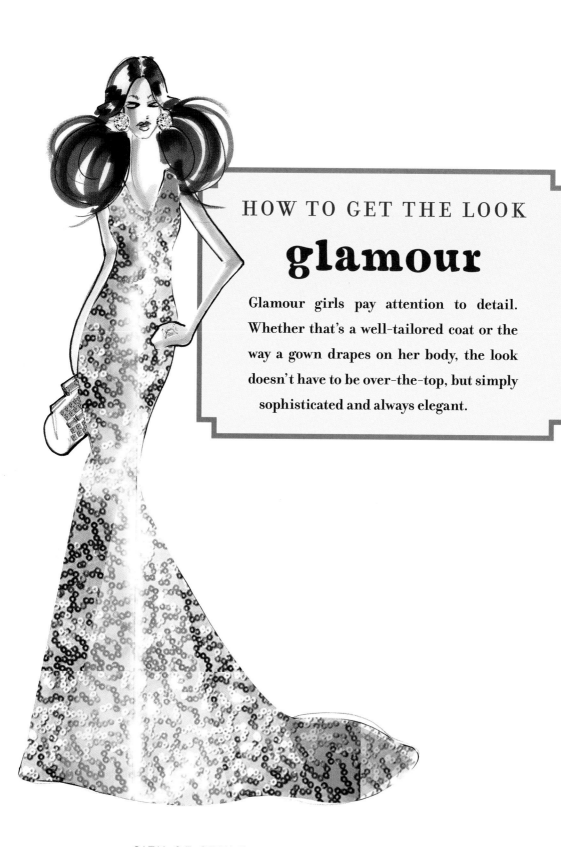

HOW TO GET THE LOOK

glamour

Glamour girls pay attention to detail. Whether that's a well-tailored coat or the way a gown drapes on her body, the look doesn't have to be over-the-top, but simply sophisticated and always elegant.

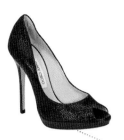

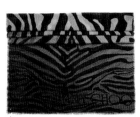

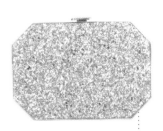

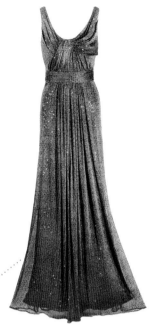

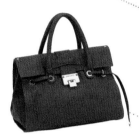

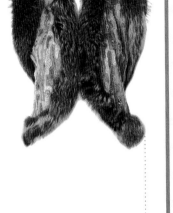

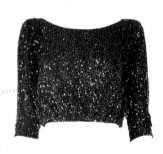

Classic high heels in black or a shimmery metallic shade add height and glamour.

Bold leopard accessories punctuate neutral basics.

A daytime bag done in a vibrant color always makes a glamorous statement.

A red carpet–worthy gown is a must for special events.

An evening bag, simple or embellished, is key for elegantly stowing necessities.

Sequins work anytime when tempered with dark denim or tailored basics.

Flare-leg denim in a saturated solid shade adds drama to a daytime look.

Classic red lipstick gives even the simplest ensemble a sexy pop of color.

Fur-trimmed outerwear always adds a dose of luxury to any look.

Shiny baubles (real or costume) are a must for any glamour girl.

Oversized sunglasses are the ultimate paparazzi shield, plus they top any look with just the right amount of drama.

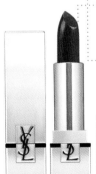

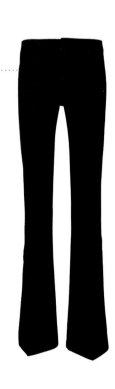

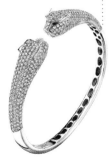

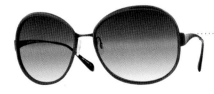

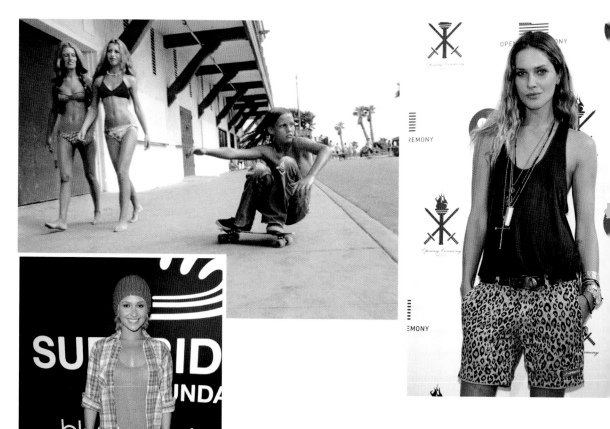

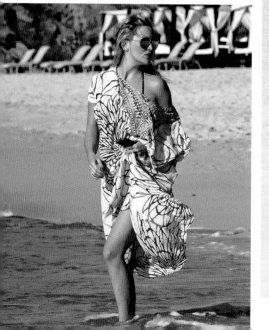

CLOCKWISE FROM TOP LEFT: Hugh Holland, *Sidewalk Surfer*, in Huntington Beach, 1976. Model **Erin Wasson** attends the Opening Ceremony Japan flagship store opening party in 2009, in Tokyo. **Cameron Diaz** prepares to surf on the set of the movie *Charlie's Angels* 2 in 2002, in Malibu. **Kate Hudson** vacations in Punta Mita, Mexico, in March 2011. **Hayden Panettiere** attends Bloomingdale's Santa Monica Surfrider Foundation Celebration Benefit at Bloomingdale's Santa Monica, April 13, 2011.

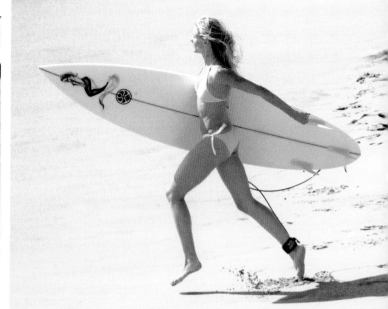

skaters and surfers

Skate is really about freedom and adaptation and constantly being confronted with obstacles you must overcome, so you have to be loose and dress loose.

—STACY PERALTA

Whether we're conscious of it or not, most of us own or regularly wear at least one item of clothing that stems from the skate or surf culture of Southern California. The look —rooted in a lifestyle evocative of freedom and fearlessness—is accompanied by a laid-back attitude. And it translates into casual clothing worn with a rough, unfinished manner and devil-may-care attitude that's been attractive not only to skaters and surfers, but to plenty of clothing companies who emulate the look in their own lines for its organic origins and unfussy approach to dressing.

The style has become popular all over the world, due in no small part to the influence of the tanned, bleached Southern California surfer and the gritty, carefree skater who are as synonymous with the city as the Hollywood sign or a palm tree–printed cup from In-N-Out Burger, and who have set the pace and core aesthetic of the style.

The relaxed demeanor, mop of sun-bleached hair, languid slouch, and golden skin of California surfers is the stuff those of us living in chilly, landlocked terrain pine for. And the rebellious, somewhat aggressive, and proudly scruffy exterior of skaters appeals to anyone who's ever enviously watched a group of kids on their skateboards careening down the street—unaffected by traffic and clearly having the time of their lives.

The common component between the two sports—and the aspect that is the most appealing to those who actually do it—is freedom. Freedom comes in the form of being disconnected from material things and instead being able to focus on and experience oneness with the environment and a connection to just the ocean or the streets and the sidewalk.

And though the two looks have a somewhat different aesthetic, Southern California skate-style was born out of what surfers wore and how they wore it.

"Skate-style really began with surfing," says retired pro skater and skate industry legend Tony Hawk. "They were trying to emulate the waves when they were flat. But as skating got more prolific people realized the potential of the urban landscape and skate-style became a mix of surf-style and punk rock. It was a more edgy look." Where surf-style has the kind of beachy component expected from a sport that takes place in the ocean, skate-style has a harder feel that comes from the influence of punk as well as being a more urban activity.

Perhaps that's the attraction of and the reason why surf- and skate-style seems to resonate with such a wide variety of people. It's not just a look and a way of life that draws thrill seekers to try surfing but also an appealing aesthetic to fashion companies everywhere, who churn out tissue-thin T-shirts and hoodies emblazoned with Southern California surf destinations, frayed denim shorts, and colorful cotton jersey dresses that convey the simplicity and long summer days associated with surfing and skating. It's the antithesis of the opulent clothing trotted down a high-fashion runway or assembled in a glossy magazine editorial, yet the organic and easy manner in which the look of skaters and surfers has evolved is undoubtedly influential and appealing to the fashion community and stylish people in general.

Because these are individual sports, skaters and surfers ride alone, developing not only signature athletic styles, but signature street styles as well. It's not just the specific clothes they wear, but how they wear them that gets noticed, sets them apart, and remains interesting.

Former pro surfer and skater turned writer/director Stacy Peralta remembers the way he and fellow surfers stood out at Venice High School during the 1970s, even when what they were wearing was exactly the same as everyone else.

"We all wore the same outfit, the Latinos, African American kids, and us surfers," he says. The look consisted of pinwale cords or Levi's, a white T-shirt with a Pendleton button-down shirt over it, and shoes called winos—two-dollar black mesh shoes with a gum sole that were typically worn by bums.

"The surfers wore everything really baggy," he says. "We carried ourselves in a slouching mentality and of course our clothes had sand and salt water on them. The Latinos pressed everything to a T and their Pendletons were buttoned to the top. The other guys didn't like us because we were surfers and looked like surfers, but it was funny because we were all wearing the same thing."

Today, the skate/surf clothing industry includes mainly logo-driven T-shirts, colorful and splashy board shorts, and printed cotton dresses that can be thrown over a bikini or worn with flip-flops. But like Peralta's simple yet individually styled look of the 70s, it wasn't always about logos and sunset-colored graphics on hooded sweatshirts.

Before the big action sports brands was influential in kick-starting the local action sports clothing industry was Jeff Yokoyama, who founded Maui and Sons in the early 80s and went on to create other brands as the sport and style evolved.

Yokoyama, an LA native and longtime surfer with a natural knack and appetite for design, embarked on what would be one of the first and most memorable surf lifestyle–centered brands to come out of the West Coast. After spending three years surfing Hawaii and then coming back to

---

simon doonan

The California beach aesthetic has had a dominant global influence for over half a century. It has a groovy sensibility, which says, "Don't take life too seriously. Why be unhappy and ambitious and type A when you can throw on a pair of Daisy Dukes, empty your head of all profundities, and head to Zuma?"

(think Hurley, Volcom, and RVCA) came around, the look surfers generally donned (which really started to take shape in the 1960s) was a uniform of white jeans, madras shirts, St. Christopher medallions, and huarache sandals that many of them traveled down to Mexico to get. Clothing was practical, simple, and free of logos except for a few companies like OP, Hobie, and local board shorts brands. Action sports lifestyle brands were not nearly the behemoth industry they are today. It wasn't until the early 80s that the commercial side of the skate/surf lifestyle started to be incorporated into clothing like we see it today.

One Southern California surfer who

Orange County to get his cosmetology license, Yokoyama noticed that the kids of the women coming through the Newport Beach salon where he worked had nothing cool to wear. Their clothing didn't reflect the beachside lifestyle they were all familiar with and definitely not the upbeat vibe of youth. He was inspired to create something for kids and teenagers that captured the lifestyle happening on the beach and made a pair of elastic waistband, madras shorts, which would be the beginning of the Maui and Sons brand.

Running the entire operation from his garage, Yokoyama created madras shorts that were a hit with teenagers because of the colorful patterns and the overall casual nature of the clothing. "I thought to myself, 'I need to supply these kids with something new and groovy,'" says Yokoyama, who from standing in the posh salon all day witnessed women wearing Norma Kamali dresses with large shoulder pads, oversize Calvin Klein blazers and Versace belt buckles and realized he could essentially do for the beach market what high fashion was doing for trend-conscious women in the 80s. The Maui and Sons circle logo with neon geometric shapes became a ubiquitous symbol throughout the 1980s, as did the overall splashy and colorful designs. He counts MTV, new wave bands like Oingo Boingo and Boy George and the thriving Southern California punk scene to be major influences in the initial look of the brand.

As the company infrastructure grew more corporate, Yokoyama became disenchanted with the mass-market turn the brand was taking, so he sold Maui and Sons and started a new line called Pirate Surf. Pirate Surf started in the early 90s and reflected the burgeoning grunge aesthetic from Seattle that was permeating the country at the time. The look of Pirate Surf was the complete opposite of Maui and Sons, dropping the neon brights for more subdued colors that were indicative of what was happening in pop culture and music at the time, translated of course for the surf lifestyle.

"We tried to make an acid-wash flannel shirt and burned holes in it by accident. There were these tiny little holes all over the shirt and we told people that it was by design, that we made the holes on purpose and everyone wanted it. That's what made the surf clothing market so bitchin' back then. No one really knew how to do it and we just capitalized on our mistakes." Pirate Surf made up to one million dollars on their acid-washed shirts, quite a feat considering this was happening before high-end, designer T-shirts were the ubiquitous staple of the fashion industry they are now.

Yokoyama would also take notice of what the surfers who rode for the Pirate Surf team were wearing and how they would tweak their clothing, many times gaining inspiration from raggedy shirts that had a sun-faded wash of color. He absorbed design ideas and inspiration from what they wore on a daily basis, whether that meant showing up fresh from the beach in shirts bleached by the sun or with the sleeves ripped right off. Yokoyama claims that it was those young surfers who were creating the trends and clothes that would be produced and put into the line. He replicated their sun and saltwater-faded T-shirts by leaving fifteen hundred shirts in his swimming pool for the chlorine to eat up the color.

The shirts were a hit with more than just local surfers and the growing contingent of people who simply wanted to look like them. Once Kurt Cobain started wearing the thin T-shirts smattered with tiny holes, the brand gained even more notoriety and was soon acquired by industry giant Quiksilver.

The happy-go-lucky nature and organic evolution of Yokoyama's surf lifestyle brands continued after Pirate Surf, but this time melded the action sports aesthetic with the then-massive trend toward all things modern and midcentury modern. "All of a sudden everything went modern and midcentury," he says. "Words like 'Scandinavian,' and 'Mies van der Rohe' were everywhere. Someone would say, 'There's this Eichler house up in Tustin. You gotta go see it.'"

Adapting to the idea that the interest of young adults was peaked by this move toward midcentury modern, Yokoyama started the Modern Amusement brand. It was another surf-inspired label, but this time with a clean, almost preppy appeal that was much different from his last venture and captured the trend at the time as well as how surfers were evolving with their own style. The look was the antithesis of Pirate Surf—clean, simple, and reduced, without the acid-washed or burned holes that were a Pirate Surf signature. The brand launched in Japan first, creating massive buzz and sales. After it was introduced in the United States and gained popularity, Yokoyama sold the company to Mossimo Giannulli (who also created the Mossimo brand) and soon departed to begin another company that he was passionate about and felt encapsulated something new, fresh, and ahead of the pulse.

He started Generic Youth in 2004 with creative input from his then-fifteen-year-old daughter. The line is carried in Yokoyama's store, Yokishop, in Newport Beach, where a tailor named Sergio makes one-of-a-kind hoodies and T-shirts from recycled fabrics. Yokoyama's daughter helped him tap into what kids were creating them-selves and interested in at the time, obviously a major source of inspiration for him in the past and a natural way of doing things that reflected the surf culture and mentality in general.

"The kids that we've been around would have blown your mind," he says. "The surf industry is about harnessing that energy again without distorting what they're doing."

Back in the 70s, when skateboarding was becoming more mainstream in Southern California, those "kids" were the Z-Boys like Stacy Peralta, Tony Alva, and Jay Adams. Peralta and his fellow Z-Boys were responsible for starting fashion trends while skating the concrete of Venice and Santa Monica—not just with their style of fluid, surflike technique but also for wearing certain items that people quickly began to emulate. "Tony [Alva] and Jay [Adams] popularized the wool fedora," says Peralta. "They started wearing them as skateboarders back in the 70s and when I released the *Dogtown* documentary in 2001, Tony was featured in it skating with a fedora on and the fedora became popular again."

Hawk's signature long blond bangs during the 80s were also a heavily emulated style element. The angular cut—which required an adequate amount of attitude to keep tossing the hair back from his face—was and still is an iconic style hallmark in the world of skate.

"I never felt pressure to be iconic or try to inspire a new look. I just liked what I liked," he says. "I liked growing my bangs in the 80s. It wasn't just punk. It wasn't just skate. [The hairstyle] just sort of represented a certain style of music and my interest in skating. And that hairstyle got copied a lot."

Style elements from the surfers and skaters of the past are consistently being referenced today. The shimmery, sun-bleached locks of hair that are synonymous with surfers have been attractive for decades and continue to inspire women, who have adopted the ombre "grown-out" look that leaves their roots several shades darker than their platinum blond tips. A pricey salon process called Balayage ensures that their hair gets an almost ombre effect of being bleached by the sun, a signature aspect of spending time on the beach and outdoors. "I used to work at the old Venice Noodle Company over on Main Street when I was seventeen," says Peralta. "Women would come over to me and go absolutely crazy for my [sun-bleached] hair."

Like a surfer's sun-kissed hair spawning salon treatments, several other fashion-related items have evolved from the practical aspects of surfing and skating. Perhaps the most ubiquitous one is the UGG boot that, starting in Australia in the 1960s, became a favorite of surfers who would shove their freezing feet into the boots right as they jumped out of the water and onto the beach. The simple shearling-lined bootie has become a sartorial staple for everyone from teenagers and housewives to Britney Spears out on a Starbucks run.

The button-front Pendleton-style flannel shirt has also served the same purpose and fallen in line as a grungy basic worn with skinny jeans and boots by celebrities off duty. Surfers throughout the 1960s and 70s wore these types of shirts all the time as a way to get warm after emerging from the ocean, especially during early morning surf sessions. And as T. K. Brimer, owner of the legendary Newport Beach surf shop Frog House puts it, "Any good surfer was up early to go surfing."

From the skaters, useful little tricks like replacing a leather belt with a less obtrusive shoelace to hold up their sagging pants became commonplace, and soon major skate apparel manufacturers built a shoelace drawstring into men's pants, which sold at mass-market street-wear stores like Tilly's.

The surf and skate aesthetic is still apparent in many clothing lines, including James Perse, Splendid, and even Alexander Wang—especially seen in his early collection staples such as supershort frayed denim cutoffs, slouchy knit beanies, and drapey T-shirts, which represented a feminized yet still gritty version of the skater look. And of course there are the locally based brands steeped in the history of both activities like Roxy, Quiksilver, Hurley, and RVCA that like Yokoyama's various labels originated in the culture of action sports and have evolved into fashion and lifestyle brands.

Skate-based footwear like Vans has become a common accessory with everyone from grade school–aged kids to older people looking to subtly add a street-wear edge to their look.

Hawk's visibility as a pro skater as well as his video games and brand of skate competitions have made him a sports figure and mogul. His clothing line sells at Kohl's, where as he puts it, "Moms in the Midwest can afford skate-influenced looks for their kids." The line is based on clothing Hawk himself wears as well as what other fashion-savvy skaters wear. Slim-leg jeans, checkered shirts, and striped hoodies are available in Hawk's clothing line for boys, ranging from toddlers to teens and proving that even for the kids who don't

orful Body Glove wetsuits and rash guards from the 80s. They cited skateboarding, surfing, and the images of photographer Glen Friedman, who documented the California skate culture scene in the 1970s and 80s, as their major inspiration that season.

The design duo, Jack McColbugh and Lazaro Hernandez, claimed to be referencing a lot of old Powell-Peralta surf films to inform their collection and told Elle.

CYNTHIA ROWLEY

The most appealing aspect of surf-style for me is the self-assuredness that's conveyed. The laid-back styles reinforce a certain level of comfort and confidence, no matter what the situation.

skate (yet), skate-style is something that's become a part of the greater fashion vernacular.

Perhaps the influence of the Southern California skate and surf culture is most apparent with brands like American Eagle Outfitters, Hollister, and Abercrombie & Fitch (which are based in the Midwest), who carry T-shirts and sweatpants emblazoned with local California surf spots or vintage-driven California surf graphics. It's a testament to how appealing the aesthetic is and how it will always represent an aspirational lifestyle.

High-end designers are attracted to the style of skaters and surfers as well. For their spring 2010 collection, Proenza Schouler turned out neon-hued tie-dye pieces reminiscent of the splashy and col-

com in a 2010 interview, "We're big fans of the early Bones Brigade stuff, the early videos of Tony Hawk, Steve Caballero, and the gang messing around on films like *The Search for Animal Chin* is still a huge reference for us. We grew up in different parts of the country, but both worshipped the guys in those videos. It was more the stylistic angle or rather, the attitude."

Designer Cynthia Rowley isn't just inspired by West Coast surf and skate culture—incorporating the sporty aesthetic into her ultrafeminine line—she has also lent her talents to Roxy, collaborating on a collection of wet suits and beachwear for the brand. "The most appealing aspect of surf-style for me is the self-assuredness that's conveyed," says Rowley. "The laid-back styles reinforce a certain level of comfort and confidence, no matter what the situation." Rowley's creations for Roxy take a retro California surf-style and add more modern design elements to, as she puts it, "honor the legacy while still creating something new."

While high-end designers are tapping into the skate and surf scene for creative stimulation, the action sports industry has simultaneously been upping their design game to embrace a more sophisticated look to clothing and accessories that continue to appeal to both the youth and the adult markets.

The action sports industry has boasted billion-dollar annual sales in the past several years due largely in part to the fact that the clothes no longer mainly consist of hibiscus floral prints and knee-length board shorts. There are still the bread-and-butter pieces like logo T-shirts and hoodies emblazoned with brand graphics, but over the past decade, the action sports industry has developed items that are more trend driven and fashion forward, while still keeping the easy, nonseasonal California lifestyle in mind. The lines between skate, surf, and casual beachwear have blurred a bit into more of a street-wear look. Skaters' pants are tapered, board shorts are shorter, and the women's clothes are meant for layering and usually adorned with some kind of trendy and edgy detail like studs or angular 80s-style print.

The overtly beachy or baggy skater look that many Southern California action sports brands like Quiksilver, Roxy, DC, and Etnies once produced has blended with second-skin jeans, supershort denim shorts, vintage-inspired outerwear and bags, and footwear that follows designer collections and runway trends.

But even as these lines gravitate toward a cleaner and more fashion-forward aesthetic, the soul and heritage of their roots remain, mixing the core of the Southern California skate and surf lifestyle with trend-driven pieces for a look that was created here, but can be found in closets all over the world.

TRINA TURK

There is the option to be in the mountains, the city, the beach, or the desert within a short distance, so you end up with this closet full of clothes where you're ready for just about anything.

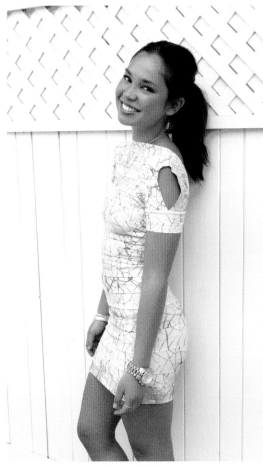

Oleema Miller

Oleema Miller, Kalani Miller

Name: OLEEMA MILLER   Hometown: san clemente, ca

Occupation: designer

How would you describe your style?

I would describe my style as laid-back, relaxed, and chic.

What are your go-to pieces and your favorite item in your closet?

My go-to pieces are always white T-shirts. And you'll rarely find me without my silver shark tooth necklace that I had made in Bali.

What is the last thing you bought?

The last thing I bought is actually not a clothing item but the most amazing vintage Moroccan wedding blanket that I got from a woman who finds them in Marrakesh marketplaces and sells them.

Who are your favorite designers?

Isabel Marant, Chloé, Stella McCartney, Helmut Lang, and Vince.

Name your signature scent?

When I do wear perfume, I love Kai's roll-on perfume (it reminds me of Hawaii!).

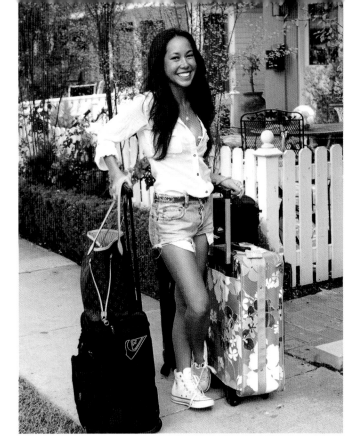

Name: **KALANI MILLER**   Hometown: SAN CLEMENTE, CA
Occupation: DESIGNER AND WORLD TRAVELER

How would you describe your style?

My style is laid-back and beach chic. I spend the majority of the year on the road, living out of a suitcase, so you have to be creative, versatile, and always have some great basics.

Who or what inspires how you dress? Who are your style icons?

My entire wardrobe is inspired by traveling, so comfy jeans and travel pants are a must. I love to pull inspirations from all over the world. And the beach inspires me, of course!

What are your go-to pieces?

My go-to pieces are a great pair of denim cutoffs and my Converse Chuck Taylors.

I think that every closet should have numerous Chucks in them . . . black, white, pink, and textured. I love them all! And no matter where I go, there are always at least three bikinis in my bag.

Name your signature scent, hairstyle, hair color, or other things you feel distinguish your style.

I love having the beachy look of salty windblown hair and the natural highlights you get from the sun, which also give your cheeks that sunny-on-the-verge-of-being-sunburned color. You just can't go wrong with the beachy look.

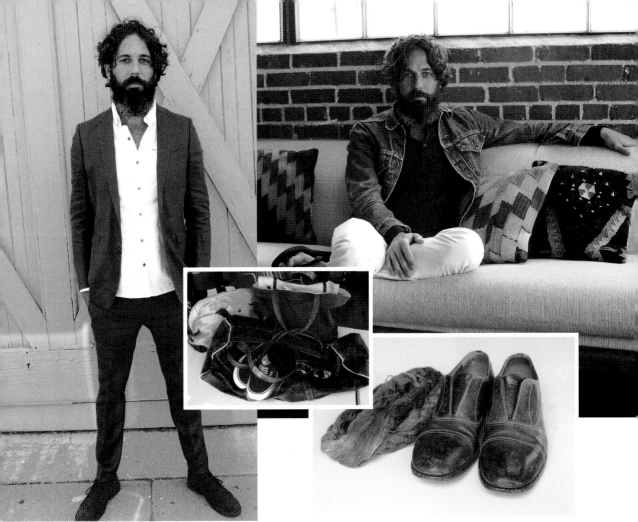

Name: JOHN MOORE   Hometown: Venice, CA   Occupation: Creative Director

How would you describe your style?

Modern coastal classic . . . always slightly disheveled.

Who or what inspires how you dress? Do you have any style icons?

My inspiration changes daily . . . the sunshine, the last song I heard, or an old photograph. Two images that come to mind are Steve McQueen and his 1956 Jaguar and Miki Dora in a sport coat with Duke Kahanamoku.

What are your go-to pieces and/or your favorite item in your closet?

My Martin Margiela shoes. Most of my closet is vintage (everything old is new again). I wear an old Levi's trucker jacket more than any other item of clothing, but I always pair it with something smart and slightly disheveled. I'm always finding beauty in imperfections.

Who are your favorite designers and your go-to places to shop?

Always vintage or my own designs I suppose. If I wear a designer, it's probably Dries Van Noten. My favorite place to shop is the Rose Bowl Flea Market, hands down.

What are your grooming habits? Do you have a signature scent?

Grooming habits? Not too many . . . just let the beard go. Does salt water have a scent?

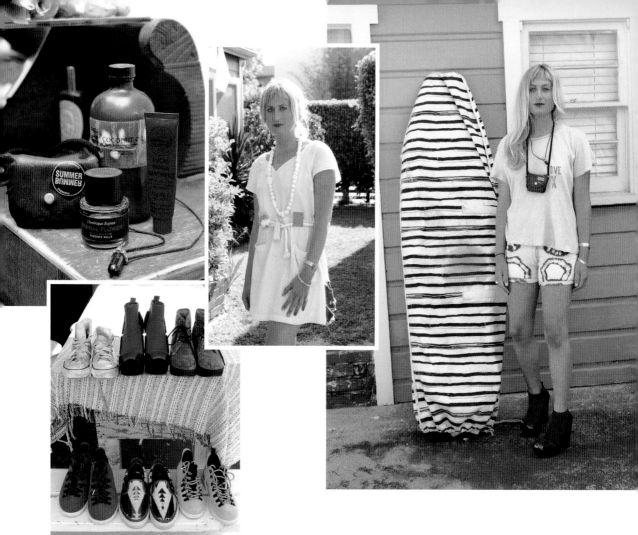

Name: **ALEXANDRA CASSANITI**

Hometown: LEUCADIA, CA, AND HONOLULU, HI   Occupation: FASHION DESIGNER

How would you describe your style?
Meticulously disheveled.

Who or what inspires how you dress? Who are your style icons?
Looking at old photos of surf culture in Australia, Hawaii, California, especially John Severson's books and photos. Surfing inspires me, so does nature and the ocean.

What are your go-to pieces?
Right now, I wear the cheesecloth shirts that I make. They are really easy to layer, and don't irritate your skin . . . I know, so nerdy! Sensitive skin! I like to layer. You never know if you are going to get cold or

hot, or spill something on yourself. This way you can take something off or rearrange.

Who are your favorite designers?
I respect so many! I like Alexander McQueen, Sonia Rykiel, Chanel, Yves Saint Laurent, Preen, Hussein Chalayan, Hermès, Henrik Vibskov, Robin Piccone, Dare Jennings, Flax, Tiffany Tuttle, Ann Demeulemeester, Mary Ping, and Acne.

What is your signature hairstyle?
My hairstyle is long, blond, and most of the time just ocean water, barely brushed.

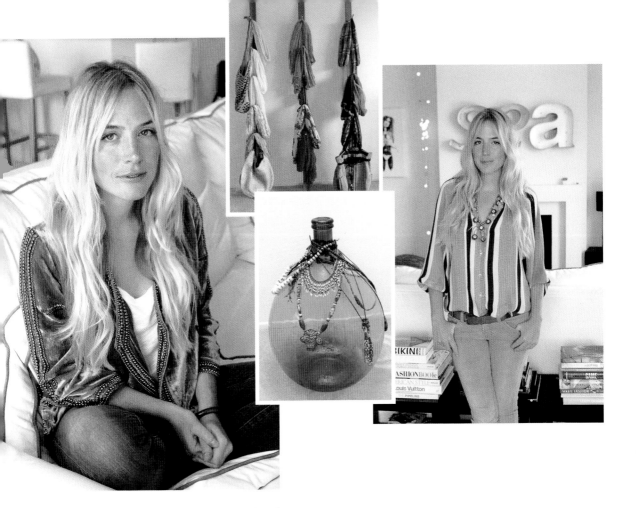

Name: **LISA PRIOLO**   Hometown: TORONTO, ONTARIO
Occupation: RETAIL CONSULTANT

How would you describe your style?
My style is a healthy mixture of West Coast, California beach vibe combined with a slightly more serious East Coast sensibility.

What are your go-to pieces and/or your favorite item in your closet? And what would you consider a signature aspect of your style?
I'm a jeans girl. J Brand is my brand of choice; I have a pair in pretty much every color as they act as the perfect blank canvas. I am also a huge fan of Tucker's smock silk blouses. I buy one each season. They are the best-fitting blouse and hang like no other. A signature aspect to my style is adding a bold focal point or a pop of color

to an outfit. I usually achieve this look with a strong piece of jewelry, a colorful vintage belt (I collect vintage Missoni belts), or a scarf.

Who are your favorite designers?
Missoni, Dries Van Noten, and Stella McCartney.

Name your signature scent, hairstyle, hair color, or other things you feel distinguish your style.
I like subtle scents. Amber oil is my favorite. I wear my hair long and tousled. It has a sun-bleached look to it with blond highlights and natural tones mixed in—a combo that matches my freckles perfectly.

Name: **CAMERON LAING**

Hometown: SYDNEY, AUSTRALIA   Occupation: MUSICIAN

How would you describe your style?

Simple yet effective.

What would you consider a signature aspect of your style?

I love the color red. I think it stands out and makes people notice you. I love my red leather jacket and my red Converse.

What are your grooming habits?

I keep my head shaved all year round. It saves a lot of time when showering.

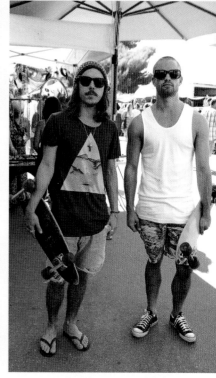

Name: **WADE OSBORN**

Hometown: SYDNEY, AUSTRALIA   Occupation: MUSICIAN

How would you describe your style?

I wear a lot of vintage and predominately button-ups, but during the summer I dress mainly for comfort.

What are your go-to pieces?

I have a phenomenal collection of Hawaiian and flannel shirts.

What is the last thing you bought?

A vintage Harley-Davidson T-shirt on Melrose.

What are your grooming habits?

Multiple shirt changes.

Wade Osborn, Cameron Laing

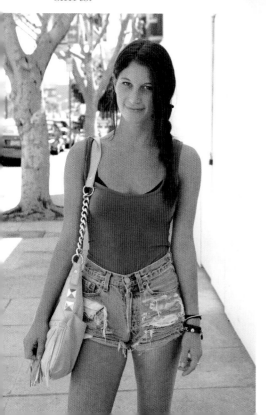

Name: **LAUREN PHILLIPS**

Hometown: LOS ANGELES, CA   Occupation: STYLIST

How would you describe your style?

I like to mix up different styles and create my own looks. Some days I feel grungy, sometimes I'm lazy and throw on a maxi and some flats, and some days I like to dress up even if I'm just going to the grocery store.

Do you have any style icons?

I am obsessed with Mary Kate and Ashley Olsen. I have followed them since I was a kid.

What is the last thing you bought?

The last item I bought was a green Marc Jacobs skirt from Wasteland.

Who are your favorite designers?

Marc Jacobs, DVF, Alexander McQueen.

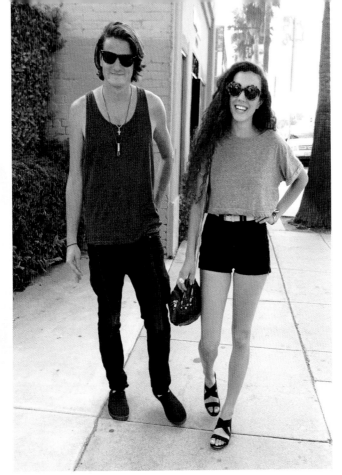

Simon Mohos, Tonya Papanikolov

Name: **SIMON MOHOS**
Hometown: TORONTO, ONTARIO   Occupation: TV HOST

How would you describe your style?
Dark, preppy, edgy.

What are your go-to pieces?
Black Cheap Monday jeans.

What is the last thing you bought?
Last thing I bought was a vintage Burberry collared sweatshirt.

Who are your favorite designers?
Andrew Buckler and Acne.

Name: **TONYA PAPANIKOLOV**
Hometown: TORONTO, ONTARIO   Occupation: PUBLIC RELATIONS INTERN

How would you describe your style?
I would describe my style as minimal with an edge.

Who are your style icons?
Ali MacGraw in *The Getaway* and Edie Sedgwick in general.

What is the last thing you bought?
Last thing I bought was my Alexander Wang black Diego shoulder bag.

Who are your favorite designers?
Favorite designers are Alexander Wang, Alexander McQueen, and Acne.

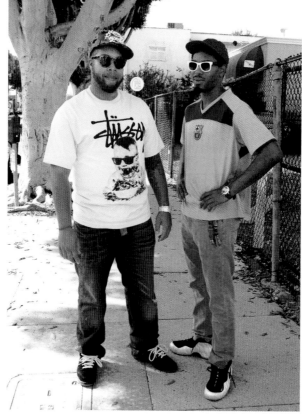

Jourdan A. Davis, Zac Davis

Name: **JOURDAN A. DAVIS** Hometown: WASHINGTON, DC
Occupation: CATERING DIRECTOR/CHEF

How would you describe your style?
I describe my style as a mixture of urban boutique brands with high-end labels.

Who are your style icons?
Kenny Burns, Ralph Lauren, and Karl Lagerfeld.

What are your go-to pieces?
Nixon timepieces, Nike Destroyer jacket, tennis shoes—all colors, brands, styles.

What was the last thing you bought?
Adidas Jeremy Scott JS Wings sneakers.

Name: **ZAC DAVIS** Hometown: WASHINGTON, DC Occupation: STUDENT

How would you describe your style?
Chill, opportunistic, random, thrifty, and resourceful.

Do you have any style icons?
Marsellus Wallace in *Pulp Fiction*.

What are your go-to pieces?
A teal shirt with bubblegum pink and blue stripes, and probably my skinny black jeans, black Vans or Nike SB sneakers.

What would you consider a signature aspect of your style?
The limitless range and versatility.

What is the last thing you bought?
Black socks with white marijuana leaves all over them—swag.

Who are your favorite designers?
Marc Jacobs, Betsey Johnson, Ralph Lauren.

What are your grooming habits?
Roll out of bed, roll up, roll out.

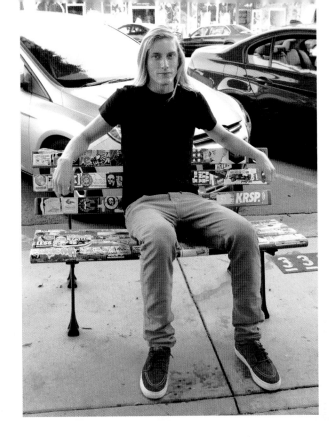

Name: XANDER MOZEJEWSKI   Hometown: HOLLYWOOD, CA
Occupation: COMMERCIAL PHOTOGRAPHER-ASSISTANT AND OCCASIONAL MODEL

How would you describe your style?
Shabby chic. I heard that on a commercial, and I love saying it.

Do you have any style icons or count any films as inspiration?
Kanye West is the biggest inspiration in my life.

What are the go-to pieces in your closet?
I have a bunch of black Calvin Klein and white Kirkland (the ones from Costco) T-shirts. That's all I wear. I have fifteen pairs of pants and more than one hundred pairs of Nikes. A signature aspect to my style is my Louis Vuitton print shoelace belt. All skaters use shoelaces for belts, and mine stands out.

What is the last thing you bought?
I just bought some Levi's Made and Crafted jeans. They are the nicest pants I've ever had. I also got the Nike Air Mags, which are replicas of the shoes Michael J. Fox wore in *Back to the Future*. They light up—it's sick.

Who are your favorite designers?
I did a shoot for *Interview* magazine where, according to the captions, I was skating in Giorgio Armani, Dior, Alexander Wang, Yohji Yamamoto, and some other super-expensive brands. I ended up ripping and messing up a lot of the stuff. I guess they're my favorite designers for letting me skate in their clothes.

What are your grooming habits? Do you have a signature scent?
I have long hair, so I wash and condition every day. I smell clean all the time—which my girlfriend hates, for some reason.

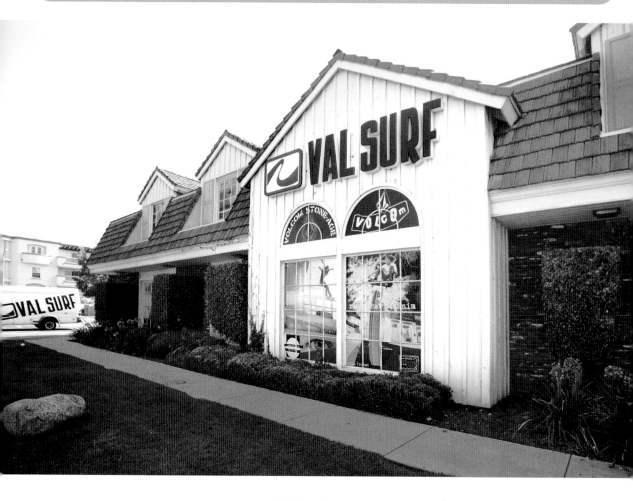

VAL SURF
4810 Whitsett Ave.
Valley Village, CA 91607
(818) 769-6977

In the early 1960s the surf craze had started in Southern California, and beaches were speckled with board shops selling surfboards to locals. But many of the kids who had caught the surfing bug lived farther inland and had to get all the way to the coast in order to buy the equipment, accessories, or apparel for their beloved sport.

Enter Val Surf, the brainchild of Bill Richards, a former record producer who,

along with his three sons, started the very first inland board shop. Located in Valley Village, California, in the San Fernando Valley, it was the first retailer to begin selling performance-level skateboards as opposed to the light and flimsy banana boards used more as toys, and it remains the oldest family-owned board shop in the world. Two of Richards's sons operate the business along with their children, and they continue to do the buying for store merchandise as well as run the day-to-day operations.

The first Val Surf store opened in 1962, years before companies like Quiksilver and Billabong surfaced and when brands such as Hobie and Ollie were the only ones creating apparel as an extension of their board line. The store's first branded apparel began with Richards's sons going down to JC Penney for plain white T-shirts and silk-screening them with their surf team competition graphics and the Val Surf logo.

They were the very first dealer of Hobie and, in the beginning, stocked the store mainly with floral shirts, huarache sandals, and cases of St. Christopher medallions, a symbol of safety and protection, something that could come in handy when facing giant waves or unforgiving pavement.

Soon, more clothing and accessories from action sports marketed brands started surfacing, and names like Gotcha, OP, and Hang Ten began to fill the store. Major companies such as Quiksilver followed and Val Surf became the first dealer to start selling the brand, as well as one of the first to carry Vans shoes from the time the popular shoe company started in 1966.

Val Surf, which now has five locations throughout the San Fernando Valley, stays focused on board sports, which in addition to skate and surf includes a massive selection of snowboarding gear and equipment. Brands like Volcom, RVCA, and Roxy, which integrate art and music into their line, are now carried in the store to accommodate the updated aesthetic of the skate/surf lifestyle.

Not only is Val Surf based in the heart of where action sports trends start and flourish, they've been around since the look and lifestyle became popular. The store was on the cusp of the trends, styles, and brands that built the industry long before it all became popular in the mainstream.

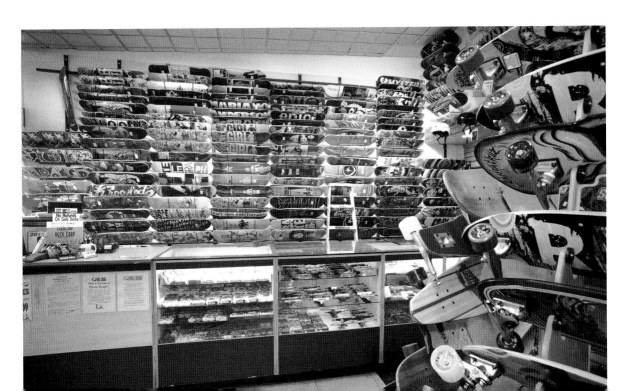

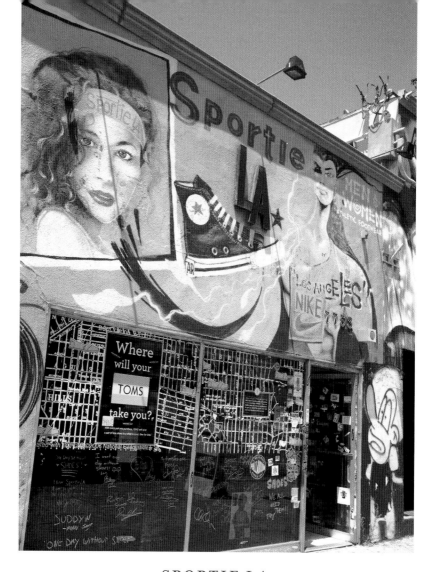

SPORTIE LA

7753 Melrose Ave.
Los Angeles, CA 90046
(323) 651-1553

Decades before sneaker heads surfaced and collecting limited edition Air Jordans became an art form, an unassuming shop on Melrose Avenue started selling sneakers of all kinds, be they traditional, trendy, or over-the-top.

It was 1985 and Isack Fadlon had just graduated from high school when his sister enticed him into starting a retail business in a storefront owned by their parents on Melrose Avenue near Fairfax Avenue. Just

teenagers, Fadlon and his sister decided to specialize in footwear and excitedly began calling all the biggest brands to place orders for merchandise. They fearlessly called major companies like Nike, Adidas, and Reebok and simply began buying things that they liked.

Twenty-five years later what started as a hobby just out of high school has turned into one the most well-known sneaker shops in the world with a reputation for having a vast selection, hard-to-find items, and interesting colors and prints other retailers dare not touch for fear that they would have too limited an audience.

Back in the 80s, Sportie LA started carrying Reebok Freestyles in every color of the rainbow from cherry red to bright yellow, when other sneaker stores were only stocking black and white.

Today, Sportie LA still stocks bright colors of Converse, limited edition collector's items, and brand reissues like the Reebok Pump or LA Gear Lights. The front of their flagship location (there are now three other stores in LA and one in San Diego) is jam-packed with nearly a hundred different brands. The sight is actually somewhat overwhelming, with every open crevice packed with some kind of sneaker.

The back of the store, however, is a respite from the sneaker madness up front. It is set up to spotlight higher-end, limited edition, or new brands in a museum-like setting. Besides having a wide range of styles, Sportie LA is also something of a sneaker archive. They sometimes buy prototypes of sneakers that were never produced by a brand, leaving them with highly valued one-of-a-kind pieces to treasure or sell to a very lucky customer.

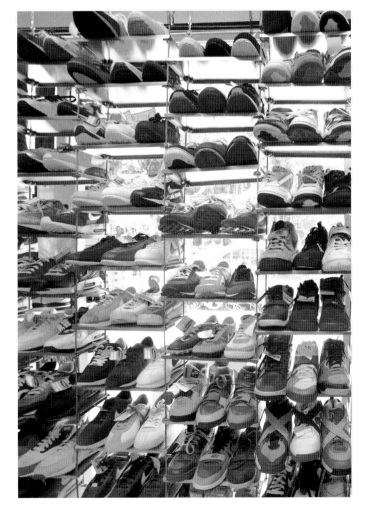

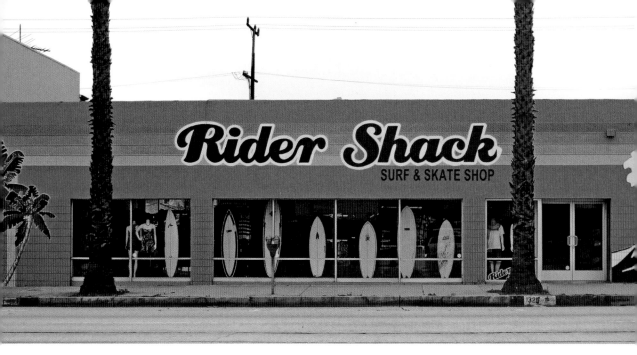

RIDER SHACK

13211 W. Washington Blvd.
Los Angeles, CA 90066
(310) 821-7873

In West LA, a few blocks from the intersection where Venice, Marina del Rey, and Culver City converge, sits Rider Shack, a 5,000-square-foot store that houses everything from wet suits and skateboards to sandals and trendy apparel from popular action sports labels. Husband-and-wife owners Jeff and Lacey Glass opened the store in 2010 to combine their passions—his, action sports and a love for surfing, hers, a knowledge of and interest in fashion and retail.

They set up the store specifically to appeal to a wide array of shoppers, everyone from the flip-flop-loving college kid or novice surfer to the seasoned surfer and skater. The store falls somewhere in between the mass board sport retailers with brand-heavy displays and a giant inventory and the old-school beach-shack-type shops that cater more to the skilled surfer and can be

somewhat intimidating for a beginner.

The atmosphere at Rider Shack is especially inviting, despite the large and airy space. The couple has always had a fondness for Mexico and created several fixtures that add to the atmosphere, like grass-topped roof facades jutting out from a few walls. They also use colorful Mexican blankets as curtains for the dressing room stalls. A long couch that looks like it was salvaged from an old car is placed right in the middle of the store among some other seats. Here, locals and friends gather and hang out, sharing the details of their early morning surf, usually accompanied by shop dog, Mako.

In addition to the homey atmosphere and mom-and-pop mentality, there is of course the merchandise—including an impressive selection of surfboards and related accoutrement. The shop carries a hundred different styles of surfboard fins and a variety of board leashes, which are housed in a back area of the store called the Board Room. A counter where skateboards are assembled and sold is also a part of the Board Room. Off of this area is an enclosed room with glass walls where the couple invites guest shapers to hand shape boards, while surf enthusiasts look on to see their skills at work.

Men's and women's clothing labels include Billabong, Rip Curl, O'Neill, and Volcom as well as Sanuk and Rainbow sandals and sunglasses from Spy, Von Zipper, Hoven, and Electric.

The Glasses plan to expand the homey feeling of the space even more during summer when movie nights will commence at the couch area, which is conveniently situated to face a large screen onto which favorite films—some surf related, of course—can be projected.

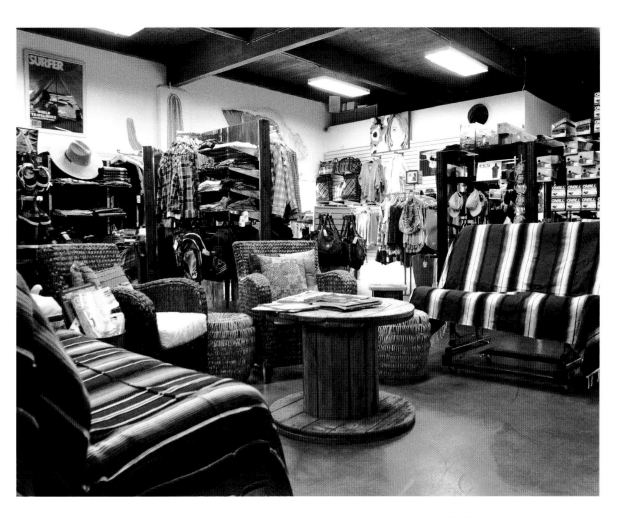

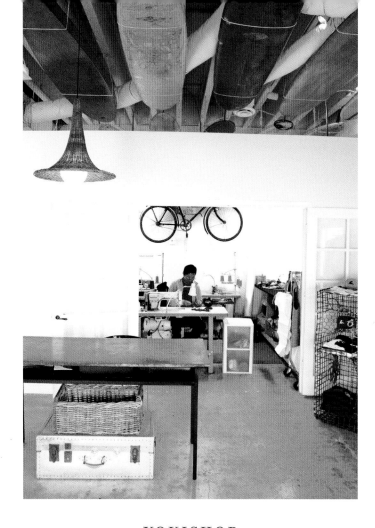

YOKISHOP
2429 West Coast Highway, Suite 102
Newport Beach, CA 92663

Action sports apparel industry veteran Jeff Yokoyama created his clothing line Generic Youth in 2004 after decades of starting and running surf-inspired clothing companies in Orange County. With his current venture, which he conceptualized with the help of his then-fifteen-year-old daughter, he abides by three basic principles: design different, make different, and sell different.

At his Newport Beach shop, Yokoyama works by this mantra and fills the space with items that speak to the surf lifestyle as well as clothing and accessories made from recycling fabrics, including old beach towels and college sweatshirts.

"When I started Generic Youth, the idea behind it was to do something different," says Yokoyama, who consulted with his daughter for fresh ideas on clothing that would feel innovative and embody a youthful spirit. They began cutting up old, perfectly worn-in sweatshirts that had faded from their once-vibrant color. The result was vintage sweatshirts repurposed into one-of-a-kind hoodies with sleeves and front panels all sourced from different places, which gave a color-blocked ef-

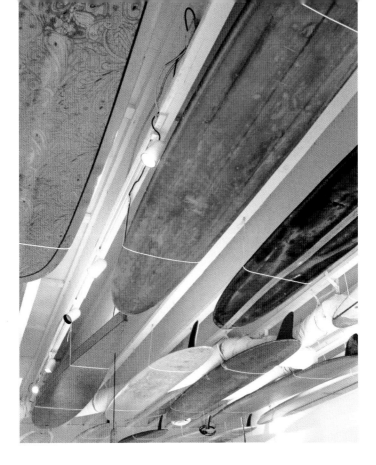

fect with the comfort and easiness of a no-brainer staple. Old keys were attached to the front as zipper pulls with the idea that each key is cut different, just like every kid is cut different.

Today, Yokoyama sells his Generic Youth label in the space as well as pieces from other lines he designs and produces, including Pidgin Orange, Mucho Aloha, and Yoki's Garden—a line of University of Southern California–branded clothing and accessories made of castaway items from the school's sports department.

Everything in the store is made by hand with the skill of an in-house tailor named Sergio, who is stationed at a sewing machine inside the space, chopping up beach towels and old sweatshirts and making new patterns to create something one-of-a-kind and decidedly surf inspired.

Board shorts are constructed from interior design fabrics Yokoyama gets from a source down the street from his shop. Cuttings from old kimonos and cashmere sweaters are repurposed as collars or piping details on T-shirts for a product that sticks to his original mantra of making clothing differently than mass-market action sports companies that are heavily branded and readily accessible.

"The youth of America is the next groove, not the CEOs," says Yokoyama about his take on creating special, one-of-a-kind, hand-crafted pieces that don't simply regurgitate a retro 1960s surf lifestyle, but rather try to capture and reflect what the free-spirited skaters and surfers he encounters are doing today. "I wanted to get back to the basics and involve the youth."

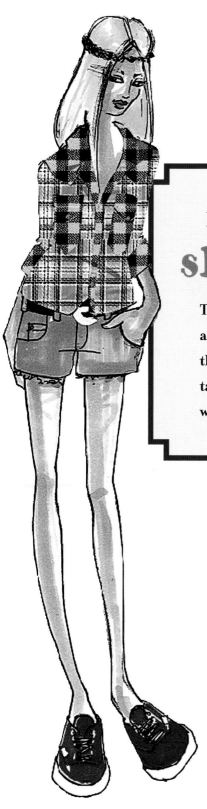

HOW TO GET THE LOOK
skate and surf

The skate and surf look is all about loose layers and casual basics that work at the beach and on the street. Denim cutoffs, tissue-thin cotton tank tops, and slouchy sweaters are always worn with an air of cool and an easy sporty style.

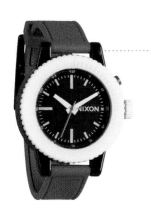

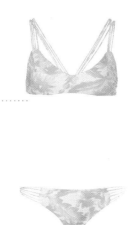

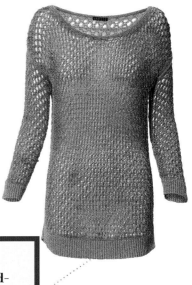

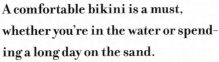

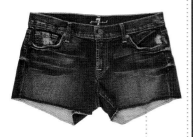

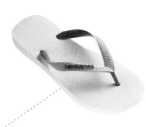

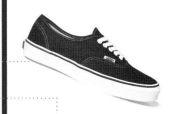

A comfortable bikini is a must, whether you're in the water or spending a long day on the sand.

Cover-ups like a loose and light sweater work well for day to night.

Comfy denim cutoffs are casual and versatile and can easily be dressed up or down.

Flip-flops are a must for running around during long summer days.

Classic Vans are a skate and surf staple.

Sunscreen will protect you for long days spent outside.

A canvas bag works well for stowing belongings on the beach.

Sporty shades provide sun protection and added style.

A waterproof watch in a vibrant shade adds a sunny pop of color.

A worn-in, vintage-inspired T-shirt is the foundation of the skate and surf look.

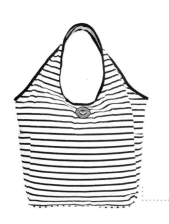

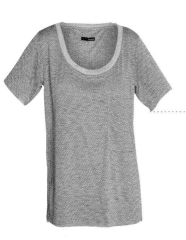

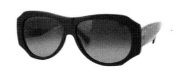

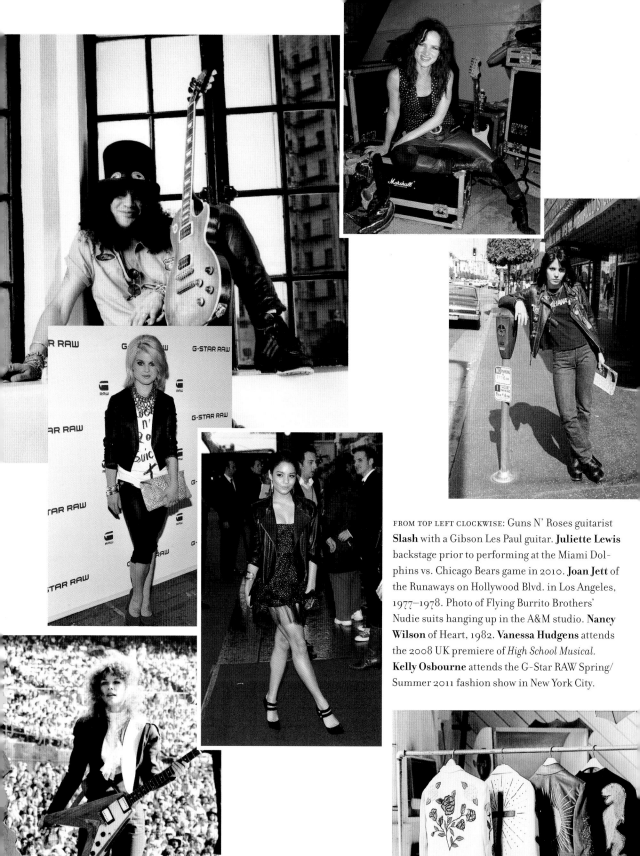

FROM TOP LEFT CLOCKWISE: Guns N' Roses guitarist **Slash** with a Gibson Les Paul guitar. **Juliette Lewis** backstage prior to performing at the Miami Dolphins vs. Chicago Bears game in 2010. **Joan Jett** of the Runaways on Hollywood Blvd. in Los Angeles, 1977–1978. Photo of Flying Burrito Brothers' Nudie suits hanging up in the A&M studio. **Nancy Wilson** of Heart, 1982. **Vanessa Hudgens** attends the 2008 UK premiere of *High School Musical*. **Kelly Osbourne** attends the G-Star RAW Spring/Summer 2011 fashion show in New York City.

rockers

The idea of rock is to break the rules and to do things your own way.

—ANN WILSON, HEART

Pinning down one specific look that embodies the culture and energy of rock 'n' roll is almost impossible. Depending on the decade and genre, rocker-style can mean anything from glitter to grunge, leather and spikes, to leopard print bodysuits, and of course the inflated, electroshock heaps of hair sported by metal bands from the 1980s.

The common denominator of the rocker look is that the rock 'n' roll lifestyle is, by nature, built on freedom and doing things your own way. And the clothing that goes along with it is an integral aspect of rock, allowing musicians to express themselves to their fullest—whether onstage or off. Between the clothes, the music, and the lifestyle, Los Angeles has long been a breeding ground for some of rock's biggest acts, whose look and sound have been both inspired by the city and influenced by the fashion landscape of LA and its unique and brazen style.

Los Angeles is a hub and a major hotbed of activity when it comes to the entertainment industry, and the music scene is no exception. From legendary music venues that pepper the Sunset Strip to the talented custom clothing designers who create pieces for the most well-known names in music, LA's rocker look is an attractive blend of universal rock 'n' roll staples (think black, leather, and well, a lot of black leather), skin (tattooed or otherwise), vintage, and an outrageous, over-the-top vibe that pulses throughout LA's entertainment industry.

From androgyny to punk to personal style that borders on performance art, LA musicians have pushed their looks to the limit, not only to reflect their colorful, open-minded surroundings but also to elevate their showmanship to the next level. For the bands that formed in L.A. during the 1970s, style was turned up full blast. Many took cues from major British rock bands as well as chose clothing based on what broadcast their attitudes and individuality the loudest. Obviously the clothes and the way they were styled often followed the lead of the music and a touring lifestyle of travel, packed shows, and, for some, all-night parties at hotels like the "Riot" Hyatt on the Sunset Strip, near music venues like the Whisky a Go Go and the Roxy.

Bands also created signature looks to help express their sound and message. Country rock crooners like Gram Parsons went to Nudies Rodeo Tailor in North Hollywood to have embroidered and embellished Western wear created for them. For rich and colorful velvet items, bands headed to the Victorian-meets-psychedelic shop Granny Takes a Trip, while others picked up on the androgynous ensembles many of the guys were sporting, borrowing their girlfriends' clothes for a slinky look that in turn inspired a slew of female rockers who admired the contrast of edgy and soft.

Ann Wilson of the band Heart says her style was influenced by what the male rock stars around her were wearing, mainly because she found their look fun and "cartoon-y." She specifically recalls seeing the members of the Rolling Stones and Led Zeppelin wearing their girlfriends' pants and fur coats. This unconventional way of dressing sparked her imagination and set the foundation for how she wanted to dress.

"It was magic when I saw Brian Jones wearing Anita Pallenberg's jacket or John Lennon wearing his girlfriend's fur coat," says Wilson. She also cites Chrissie Hynde as an influential rock-style setter, but adds that like she was doing, Hynde was also taking her cues from male rockers like the Kinks.

At the time, Wilson found men's clothes more whimsical than what was available for women, which generally consisted of skintight and/or revealing clothing. She describes her look during the early 1980s as Keith Richards on top and model and famous rock girlfriend Anita Pallenberg on the bottom. She claims that the goal was not to look prissy onstage but like a rock singer who played aggressive music, which Wilson and her sister, Nancy, accomplished with their blend of black leather, teased hair, and sky-high platform boots, tempered with flowy designer separates and lace-up corsets.

Wilson mixed garments like button-down blouses from YSL Rive Gauche with more traditional "rock" items like tight black pants or fitted vests, blending hard and soft for a romantic rock vibe. Most of her accessories came by way of fans and the tokens they affectionately threw to her onstage, items picked up while she was on tour, or things from designers who would send her their creations. The beads and jewelry fans flung to her while she was performing became a natural extension of her look. "People would toss necklaces and chains onstage and I would wind them around my ankle or wrist. Steven Tyler would just drape them around the mic," she says.

Wilson's sister, Nancy—the other half of Heart—takes a more traditional and practical approach to her onstage appearance, considering stable and supportive footwear she needs for a secure guitar-playing stance first, then dressing up from there. She has black platform ankle boots custom made in Hollywood to ensure they're just the way she likes them and takes the guitar into great consideration. But practicality does not eclipse Nancy's edgy look. She sticks to a variety of textures, including patent leather, leather, and velvet all in black. "I like to wear black—the universal rock color. Actually the absence of color is the most universal rock color, which I'm totally drawn to."

Her sense of style is not completely unlike her sister's, taking ideas from the androgynous aesthetic that was happening in rock during the 70s. "When we first started in the mid-70s, there was almost a cross-dressing thing going on," says Wilson of the fact that women were wearing men's clothes and men were wearing women's clothes. She remembers the lanky British boys who could fit easily into their girlfriends' jeans, creating the lithe and sinewy silhouette still so common with male rock stars today.

Toward the late 1970s, when punk entered the LA music sphere in a massive way, East LA native Alice Armendariz changed her name to Alice Bag and formed the punk band the Bags. Armendariz's onstage style took traditional hard rock edges and mixed them with chola-style makeup and a sexy, boundary-pushing punk aesthetic. She found the originality and creativity of punk appealing, not just for the music, but also because it valued invention and deconstruction, something Armendariz claims definitely influenced her fashion choices.

Several years before Madonna would emerge onstage wearing a bra with a crinoline skirt, Armendariz and other female punk rockers layered bras and corsets over clothing. To get the pieces for her playful and revealing stage outfits, Armendariz frequented Frederick's of Hollywood on Hollywood Boulevard, where she picked up fishnets, garters, and her favorite pair of fur-trimmed, gray suede ankle boots.

"Our style was colorful and cinematic," she says. "New York punk had that black leather jacket thing going on. That was a little too serious for me. LA had a tongue-in-cheek attitude toward fashion." She cites the movie and entertainment industry of LA as a massive influence on the way she and other punk band members dressed, saying that being playful and fun with their clothing was part of the territory, especially in LA. "We weren't afraid to look ridiculous and had an attitude of 'if you think *that's* outrageous, get a load of *this*!' I still see styles in fashion magazines today and with performers like Lady Gaga, that echo some of the things we were doing in 1977."

Pamela Des Barres was no stranger to this outlandish sense of style. In fact, she famously wore some pretty extreme getups as arguably one of the most well-known groupies and band muses of her time. For Des Barres, fashion was about turning heads, breaking boundaries, and shaking things up—a way of doing things not unlike Gaga and other pop music performers of today.

"I dressed so people would look at me," says Des Barres. She and her group of fellow teenage girlfriends would hit vintage stores around town, stretching their dollar fifty to buy dresses, tablecloths, and doilies from the 1930s and reworking them into minimal, often sheer, and always fabulously creative frocks that were just sturdy enough to dance in.

Des Barres and her group, the GTOs, danced with bands like Three Dog Night, Love, and the Flying Burrito Brothers, and caught the audience's attention with their eccentric and revealing outfits. "We were half naked most of time, but we also wore the most incredible clothes." Des Barres and her crew wore over-the-top ensembles comprised of pieces like silk velvet dresses with shirring on the sleeves, sheer flowered chiffon dresses, velvet cloaks, and capes. They also made dresses out of tablecloths and punctu-

JOHN ESHAYA

LA girls aren't afraid to mix it up! They can put together thrashed denim shorts with a hippie top and a Chanel bag. By day she might be in classic flats and boyfriend or vintage jeans, but for dinner she's in cage heels and black skinny jeans.

ated their outfits with feather boas and incredibly teased-up hair. "I'd even glue sequins all over my face in patterns," she recalls. "That's what Frank [Zappa, who produced the GTO's first and only album] loved about us. He liked the way we were living. We were actually performance artists before the term existed."

Des Barres may not have spent as much time onstage as she did off, but it's clear that she still embodied LA rock 'n' roll with her wild clothing and energy. The idea of performance art meeting rock that Des Barres and the GTOs demonstrated in LA decades ago still thrives today among performers like Lady Gaga, Katy Perry, and Nicki Minaj. While these current-day acts may be more pop than rock, the concept and motivation arises from the same place it did for musicians and groupies of the past, who harnessed their passion for music and the scene surrounding it by expressing themselves with the most extreme looks they could put together at the time.

In addition to creating her own outrageous ensembles—one of Des Barres's standout looks includes painting herself entirely green, wearing a green bikini with parsley sewn all over it, and even sporting what she calls a "parsley afro"—Des Barres also found that custom making Western-style shirts for the musicians she adored was another way to get closer to them. She created around fifty shirts, which she sewed from scratch and then hand embroidered and embellished with personal touches. The purple button-down shirt she made for her friend Gram Parsons had delicate vines and leaves running down the front and a sweet GP on the upper left-hand corner. A ratty tag with the words "Hand sewn by Miss Pamela" is stitched into each of her creations.

Besides the clothing Des Barres made for the musicians she adored, she also utilized her provocative outfits to get their attention. One night when she went to see Waylon Jennings perform, she simply wore panties that said "Hollywood" across the backside, garter belts, seam stockings, high heels, and a bra. "This was way before Madonna, thank you very much. And that's how I got Waylon one night. I dressed like that, sat right in front of the stage and tossed flowers to him onstage." She adds that Jennings was so distracted by her appearance that he kept forgetting the words to his songs.

Another hot ticket on the LA music scene at the time was Evita Corby, who started dating James Williamson, guitar player of the Stooges, when she was just a teenager. Corby moved in with the band above the Sunset Strip while they recorded their album *Raw Power*, which was on David Bowie's then record label. She was immediately immersed in the adventure, energy, and style of the time and setting and naturally started dressing both herself and her rock star friends in homespun, but nevertheless outrageous clothing.

Corby's personal style was influenced by the flower children she saw at love-ins at Griffith Park—think denim, lace, and moccasins—the leather and embroidery detail male rockers of the time were wearing, and a tinge of the British music scene's psychedelic-Victorian aesthetic. Corby's interest in clothing and knack for embroidery segued into helping her friends—most of whom were rock stars—dress in unique and custom-made pieces most often designed by her and made by Glen Palmer, the British tailor who was stationed at the LA outpost of Granny Takes a Trip.

It was common practice for the girlfriends of the bands to make all their clothes back then. "I wanted to look a certain way. The guy I was dating wanted to look a certain way. I just bought the fabric and had the clothes made at Granny's. I was a part of the scene and I was creative. I could help people get their look and their style," says Corby.

She would commission Palmer to create clothes for both herself and bands out of leopard or zebra print or lush purple velvet. Making clothes was in a way essential to Corby and her rocker pals, because at the time they were hard pressed to find pieces outrageous and personal enough at an off-the-rack store.

Between designing clothing, Corby managed the VIP area of the Roxy, which suited her passion for both music and style. It also gave her front-row 24/7 access to the greatest bands that came through LA and played stages on the Sunset Strip at the time. "I got to go to sound check to make sure all the equipment came in," says Corby. "It was just like *Almost Famous*. That movie was so realistic I can't even tell you. We were muses for the bands and they wanted us around."

While a lot of the rock 'n' roll clothing at the time was being created by girlfriends and groupies, there were also a number of legendary designers and influential stores in Los Angeles that were responsible for a vast amount of memorable pieces, worn by everyone from Elvis to Elton John. Whether they were looking for a country influence or a flashy set of giant platform shoes, people had a variety of places to score unique, off-the-wall looks to reflect their rock personas.

Granny Takes a Trip opened its doors on London's King's Road in 1966 and garnered attention for its anti–Carnaby Street aesthetic and focus on Victorian flourishes and vintage clothing. By the mid-70s a West Coast outpost of the store had opened on Doheny Boulevard in West Hollywood, and it quickly became the go-to place for anyone who wanted wild patterns, plush velvets, and altogether interesting and colorful creations. Glen Palmer, a tailor from London, executed many of the suits, shirts, and jackets. "Glen had the best eye and best ideas cause he was a rocker from London," says Corby, who collaborated numerous times with Palmer on custom-made pieces for her musician friends. By the time Granny Takes a Trip made its way to Los Angeles and changed hands from its original owners, it had evolved into a retailer of more flashy pieces sporting glitter and rhinestones, which made perfect sense in Hollywood. The LA store closed by 1977 as the glam rock and glitter aesthetic faded and punk and metal settled in. But this iconic store made its mark both on the music business and on rocker-style.

Nudie Cohn, also known as Nudie the Rodeo Tailor, made custom suits, hats, boots, and belts for the biggest names in country music since opening his North Hollywood shop in 1947. His legendary store (which shuttered in 1994) has been graced by everyone from Elvis (for whom he designed the memorable gold lamé suit), Johnny Cash (whose signature look as the "man in black" was solidified by the six bespoke suits made for him by Nudie) to country rock singer and the first person to play around with custom embellishment and inject symbols from the drug culture and other forms of debauchery into the jackets made for him by Nudie, Gram Parsons. Parsons donned jackets with needles, pot leaves, and naked women as did Sneaky Pete, the slide guitarist for the Flying Burrito Brothers, who sported a large pterodactyl on one of his jackets. Bands like the Rolling Stones and the New York Dolls followed the lead of the Flying Burrito Brothers, visiting Nudie's store when they rolled through LA in order to get something custom made.

Nudie's Western-inspired wear was in a league of its own, encompassing more than just pearl-button flap pockets and leather cowboy boots. There was a certain flair that attracted musicians who knew they could have something personal, flamboyant, and totally original. More recently, Ben Harper began collecting and wearing colorful and heavily embellished pieces from Nudie, no doubt for the showstopping look, but also most likely in homage to the great country rock crooners and rock legends of decades past.

Nudie the Rodeo Tailor and his North Hollywood shop may no longer be around, but Manuel Cuevas, his former employee and protégé, has carried on making the custom Western wear that remains popular with rock stars and country crooners. Cuevas worked with Nudie for fourteen years, creating clothing for Mick Jagger, Keith Richards, and Gram Parsons. He made the white suit that Parsons famously donned on the Flying Burrito Brother's *Gilded Palace of Sin* album, spending months with Parsons while he instructed Cuevas as to precisely what he wanted depicted on the suit. "Gram worked a lot on that suit and contributed to it. It was three months before we thought it was a go," says Cuevas.

Cuevas eventually set up his own shop in Los Angeles, where he continued to create custom-made clothing for musicians, no matter how controversial their requests were. "The press gave me a lot of grief back then," says Cuevas, who in 1989 moved to Nashville where he still makes clothing, boots, belts, and hats for the biggest country stars and musicians of today. "They'd ask, 'How do you dare to put pot leaves on jackets?' Then came Mick and Keith and they asked if I could put pictures of human organs on their clothes. I thought, 'What the heck? I can do whatever I want.' It was something new and people should express themselves."

When the glitter era arrived in Los Angeles, shoe heights rocketed into outrageous platforms and had women flocking to Fred Slatten's shoe store to get off the ground and gain some serious height and bling.

It wasn't just the glitter critters hitting up Flipper's Roller Disco and Rodney Bingenheimer's English Disco who were shod in the sky-high heels. Slatten made heavily embellished, colorful, and hand-painted platform shoes—some with real goldfish in the wedge heels—for Cher, Carol Burnett, Diana Ross, Kiss, Bianca Jagger, Bette Midler, and Elton John.

Each of these designers marked pivotal fashion moments within LA's vibrant music culture and created a legacy of unforgettable style that cemented musicians' sound and look. People like Guns N' Roses guitarist Slash created their own signature style that remains constant and influential today. By embracing the iconic sartorial staples of rock and blending them with pieces that reflected his laid-back personality, Slash developed a signature style that has become as recognizable as his sound.

"I pretty much have the same style now that I've always had," he says, and cites a simple combination of T-shirts and jeans or leather pants as definite go-tos. But he recognizes his top hat and conch shell hatband to be a real fashion statement.

Slash always considered himself a "hat guy" but could never land on the right style to suit him. One day, during the mid-1980s, he was walking down Melrose Avenue and spotted a top hat in the window of a store called Retail Slut that he felt reflected his style and personality. Low on money at the time, Slash nonchalantly strolled into the store and plopped the top hat onto his head, and then just as easily walked out of the store. Down the street at a boutique called Leather & Treasures, he spied a conch shell belt that he also stole and then cut and wore the belt on the hat as a hatband. "Later that night we played the Whiskey," he says. "That was 1985."

Rock stars like Slash formed their individual sense of style by finding and wearing things they naturally gravitated to. Those who wanted some assistance in developing their looks turned to designers like Henry Duarte, who made custom rock clothing for bands like Alice in Chains and Soundgarden.

In 1998, Duarte opened an atelier and shop that catered exclusively to the rock'n'roll aesthetic at Sunset Plaza in West Hollywood, where rockers and anyone who just wanted to look like one could come in for lace-up leather pants or a bespoke skinny Beatles-style suit. Major acts like Duran Duran, Tears for Fears, Smashing Pumpkins, Michael Hutchence of INXS, Billy Idol, Metallica, and Def Leppard walked through the doors of Duarte's studio to get outfitted for onstage ensembles or just everyday wear, which was still of course relatively extreme.

A milestone in Duarte's rock designs was a pair of leather pants that inspired not only him but also a handful of notable names in the music world. The pants were vintage North Beach leather and given to him by Slash. Lenny Kravitz saw them on Duarte and asked him to make a pair like them for him. He also made a supertight leather shirt with horn buttons going down the front to go with the pants and claims that every rock guy who saw it immediately wanted one. Duarte went on to make the leather pants for everyone from Robert Plant to Sheryl Crow and Melissa Etheridge.

While Duarte tackled a more traditional-yet-tough rock'n'roll aesthetic, LA designer Rick Owens was incorporating punk and goth into his creations. Owens started his career in Los Angeles and has since moved to Paris, though he remembers his early days of drawing up stark contrasts between the dark clothing he created and the sunny Southern California sky.

"My clothes were undoubtedly inspired by LA," says Owens, who was attracted by the contrast between the dark underground music scene and the sunshine of the city. Owens also referenced Hollywood costume designers like Adrian and Travis Banton in his clothing, saying, "I was inspired by the big Hollywood costume designers from the glamorous 30s. I just did a worn black leather and old T-shirt version of them." In a sense it was LA-style coming full circle—Old Hollywood mixed with the current-day Hollywood rock scene—resulting in a unique aesthetic that catapulted Owens to be one of the most influential avant-garde designers working today.

Whether it's goth, punk, or a good old hard-hitting rock look, rocker-style has been translated in LA to encompass a harmonious mix of freedom, optimism, and the omnipresent entertainment industry, infused of course and made even more fascinating by the city's rich and vibrant music past.

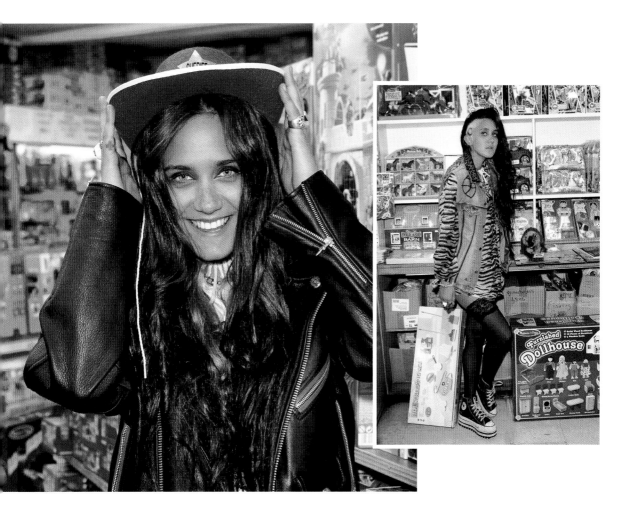

Name: **JESSE JO STARK** Hometown: MALIBU, CA
Occupation: MUSICIAN AND DESIGNER

How would you describe your style?
  Playful and instinctive.

Who are your style icons?
  Cher and the Spice Girls are my style icons.

What are your go-to pieces in your closet? And what would you consider a signature aspect of your style?
  My favorite items in my closet right now are my creepers, my platform sneakers, my "ass shorts," and my monster hair clips. My signature style is thigh-highs and brightly colored hair.

What is the last thing you bought? And what is your must-have piece of clothing right now?
  The last thing I bought was a kimono on eBay and my must-have is my cutoff vintage "Buckwheat" T-shirt.

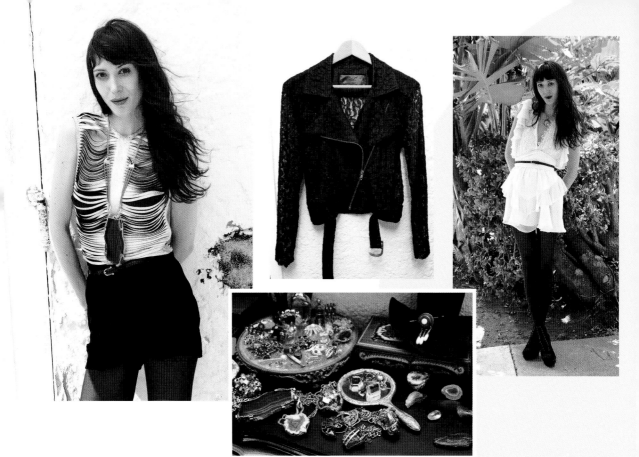

Name: **MICHELLE LAINE**   Hometown: LOS ANGELES, CA
Occupation: DESIGNER OF JEWELRY AND ART-BASED CONCEPTUAL WEAR

How would you describe your style?
Sophisticated but never polished. I'm all about putting different fashion periods and cultures together and letting them co-alesce. For example, geometric minimal-ism meets belle epoque lace, mythological neogoth revival meets embellished zulu tribal warrior, grunge rock/boho festival chic meets sleek art deco silhouettes.

Who or what inspires how you dress?
I am influenced by everything from ma-chinery and obscure mechanical compo-nents of engineering, art, and films such as *Blow-Up*, *Easy Rider*, **and** *La Dolce Vita*, **all** the way to conceptual furniture, interior design, and architecture.

What are your favorite items in your closet?
I would say my lace motorcycle jacket, high-waist velvet hot shorts, my couture cashmere cape, and all of my handmade oversized deconstructed jewelry.

What is the last thing you bought?
I just added a pair of Cuban-heeled packer boots to my already overcrowded collection of Victorian booties.

Who are your favorite designers?
Alexander McQueen, Proenza Schouler, Nicolas Ghesquière, Balmain, Ann De-meulemeester, Alexander Wang, Erick-son Beamon, Delfina Delettrez.

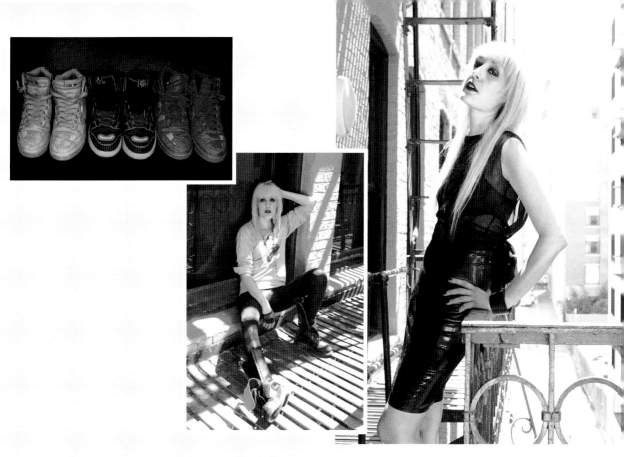

Name: IRENE URIAS   **Hometown:** LOS ANGELES, CA
Occupation: VANITY SPECIALIST

How would you describe your style?
Pit bull with a diamond collar. Chic-
tough-realness.

Who or what inspires how you dress?
Nightlife vampires. Fashion eccentrics.
People who don't believe their own hype
because they are too busy living it.

Who are your style icons?
Edina Monsoon and Patsy Stone.

What are your go-to pieces and/or your
favorite item in your closet?
Well, I'm going through a big vintage fur
phase right now. So these days I pair a fur
coat or fur accessory with everything I
wear. I have a collection of sneakers that
would make any sneaker head salivate.
Sometimes I like to turn heads in an
all-black outfit complimented by a pair of
flashy Nikes or throwbacks.

Who are your favorite designers?
It's Lacroix, Sweetie! as well as Yves Saint
Laurent, Alexander Wang, Maison Martin
Margiela, Thierry Mugler, Alexander Mc-
Queen, Rodarte, and anything Versace.

Name your signature scent, hairstyle, hair
color, or other things you feel distinguish
your style.
I think growing up in Southern California
and being under a blanket of smog at all
times has messed up my body's chemistry.
Women's perfumes don't work on me. Unisex scents like CK One are the only things
that stick. Being a hairstylist, my hairstyle and color always change. I'm going
through my big Blond Ambition moment
right now and loving it.

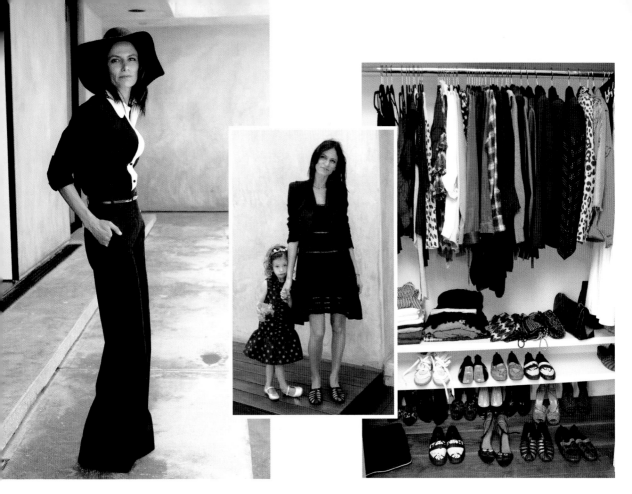

Name: MARYAM MALAKPOUR   Hometown: LOS ANGELES, CA
Occupation: FASHION CONSULTANT, STYLIST, DESIGNER

How would you describe your style?
My style is pretty much simplified classic with a "French-style" twist. There is always a bit of rock'n' roll added to the twist!

Who or what inspires how you dress?
My inspirations are often from musicians, performers, artists, and 60s French films.

What are your go-to pieces and/or your favorite item in your closet? And what would you consider a signature aspect of your style?
Skinny black jeans, a long black dress from the Row, a black leather jacket from Thomas Wylde, white T-shirts from the Row, and Isabel Marant, a Chanel bag, and Newbark flat loafers.

What is the last thing you bought? And what is your must-have piece of clothing right now?
A large-brim hat from Rodarte for Opening Ceremony. My must-have piece of clothing is a string body suit from Wolford, perfect for all the lace and sheer summer dresses!

Name your signature scent, hairstyle, hair color, or other things you feel distinguish your style.
I have two scents that I love: Tuberose from L'Artisan Parfumeur and L'Ombre from Diptyque. My hair is at a medium length, sometimes shaggy and sometimes wavy. Even if it's sleek, it's still a little bed head and never perfectly brushed.

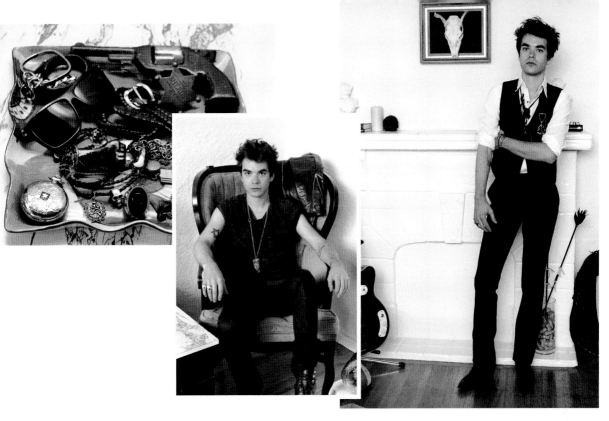

Name: **YVES BERLIN**   Hometown: ST. LOUIS, MO   Occupation: MUSICIAN

How would you describe your style?
My style is affected by my moods, so it changes frequently. I like to juxtapose vintage pieces with contemporary design.

Who or what inspires how you dress? Do you have any style icons or count any films as inspiration?
Music inspires me most definitely, 1960s Bob Dylan and the 1970s punk aesthetic of anything goes. I love the 1950s greaser mixed with my own twisted vision of a California miner during the 1800s gold rush.

What are your go-to pieces and/or your favorite item in your closet?
My go-to piece is my vintage Dior black button-down. I bought it at American Rag ages ago and have worn it to shreds. Black jean jacket with black leather sleeves, and black silk double-breasted three-piece suit that were both custom made for me.

And what would you consider a signature aspect of your style?
Black.

What is the last thing you bought?
Vintage black winkle-picker shoes with studs on them at the Melrose Trading Post flea market.

Who are your favorite designers and your go-to places to shop?
I love Endovanera, Costume National, Acne, Alexander McQueen, and Vivienne Westwood. And my girlfriend (she doesn't sell menswear) but she does custom pieces for me, and they are essential to my wardrobe. Some of my favorite places to shop in LA are Maxfield, American Rag, Confederacy, Filth Mart, and some secret vintage spots that I can't reveal.

Do you have a signature scent?
I don't have one. I let the musk of California be my scent.

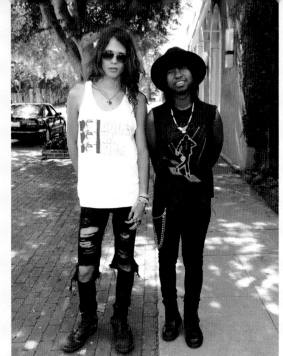

Jacob DeKat

Prince Chenoa

Name: JACOB DEKAT   Hometown: NEW YORK, NY AND LOS ANGELES, CA
Occupation: PHOTOGRAPHER AND MAGAZINE EDITOR

How would you describe your style?
A mix of grunge, punk, and glam.

Do you have any style icons or count any films as inspiration?
Jim Morrison, Mick Jagger in *Performance*.

What are your go-to pieces?
Leather, flannels, and jewelry.

What is the last thing you bought?

A snakehead necklace at the flea market in Pasadena.

Who are your favorite designers?
I love Vivienne Westwood, especially from back in the day.

What are your grooming habits?
Swimming in the sea.

Do you have a signature scent?
Rose oil.

Name: PRINCE CHENOA   Hometown: NEW YORK, NY AND LOS ANGELES, CA
Occupation: CREATIVE DIRECTOR

How would you describe your style?
Native rock.

Do you have any style icons?
Prince.

What would you consider a signature aspect of your style?
My hats, I love hats. It's the one thing I'm never without.

What's the last thing you bought?

A vintage tan suede fringe jacket from the Rose Bowl Flea Market in Pasadena.

Who are your favorite designers?
Alexander Wang and mostly flea market stuff.

Do you have a signature scent?
I love Tom Ford Tobacco Vanille. It's such a wonderful smell.

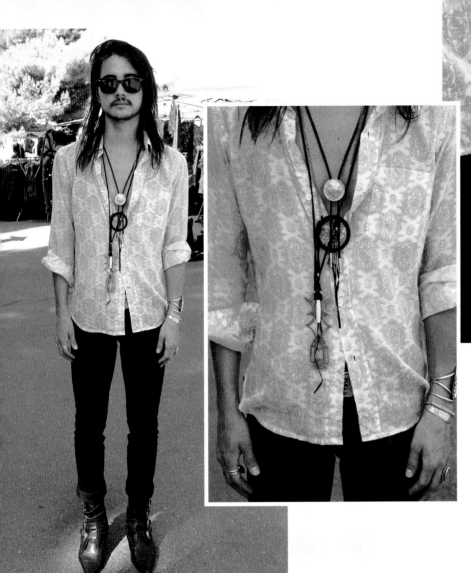

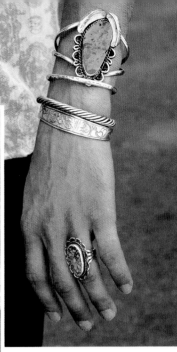

Name: DANIEL JAMES RESCH   Hometown: PHILLIPSBUrG, NJ
Occupation: PHOTOGraPHer

How would you describe your style?
I guess it would be a mix of 60s garage, psychedelic, and punk.

Who are your style icons?
Syd Barrett, Sky Saxon, Stiv Bators.

What are the go-to pieces in your closet?
My go-to pieces would be a ripped-up T-shirt or a thin button-up. My favorite item would be my vintage Stones tour shirt.

What would you consider a signature aspect of your style?
A signature aspect of my style would be music.

What is the last thing you bought?
Last thing I bought was a pair of skinny jeans.

Who are your favorite designers?
Levi's, April 77, Pendleton

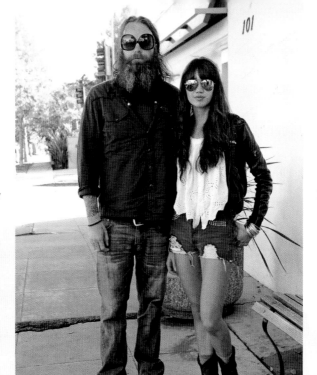

Joseph Holiday

Nalani

Name: **JOSEPH HOLIDAY**　Hometown: FREEHOLD, NJ
Occupation: MUSICIAN AND PRODUCER

How would you describe your style?
Pretty simple. I think I have been wearing jeans, black T-shirts, and boots every day for years. That never goes out of style.

Do you have any style icons or count any films as inspiration?
Mostly musicians with great style, like Nick Cave.

What are your go-to pieces and the favorite item in your closet?
I have a closet full of black T-shirts. But my favorite item would be this black corduroy mod-looking coat with a huge stiff collar, which I bought from this mod shop in London.

What is the last thing you bought?
A stars-and-stripes tank top from a thrift store in Brooklyn.

Name: **NALANI**　Hometown: WAIMANALO, HAWAII
Occupation: PART-TIME STUDENT, FULL-TIME RABBLE-ROUSER

How would you describe your style?
Cheeky yet dangerous.

Who are your style icons?
I love Joan Jett with her "F the Haters" vibe.

What is your favorite item in your closet?
My three-dollar, side-of-the-street-purchase-in-Milwaukee combat boots.

Neither rain nor snow nor sleet nor hail will stop those bad boys.

What is the last thing you bought?
These black cowboy boots I'm wearing. A ten-dollar thrift store score.

Who are your favorite designers?
I'm in love with Jeffrey Campbell wedges.

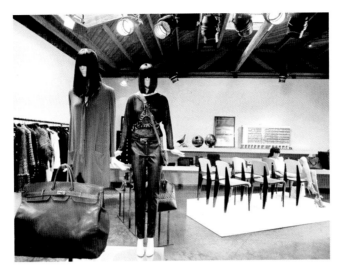

MAXFIELD
8825 Melrose Ave.
Los Angeles, CA 90069
(310) 274-8800

In the middle of West Hollywood's most posh stretch of shops, restaurants, and hair salons is Maxfield. With a sleek gray exterior, long horizontal windows, and three large concrete Roger Herman sculptures near the store's entrance, the 7,000-square-foot concrete building stands out among the light and airy structures that neighbor it.

Owner Tommy Perse opened Maxfield (originally called Maxfield Bleu) in 1969. Aside from founding Maxfield and being credited with introducing lines such as Comme des Garçons and Yohji Yamamoto to the West Coast in the 1980s, Perse is also father to California lifestyle and chic loungewear designer James Perse.

The interior of Maxfield is unlike anything in Los Angeles and perhaps the world. The store, which Karl Lagerfeld has ranked as one of his favorite shopping destinations, is filled with avant-garde and intensely edgy items from designers like Rick Owens, Thomas Wylde, and Gareth Pugh. Strapless woven leather dresses, shimmery silver-and-black bouclé jackets, skull-printed silk caftans, and cases of vintage jewelry are displayed among stone gargoyles, crocodile leather trunks, and vintage Hermès Birkin bags. Offbeat objects that add a curiosity shop kind of feel to the location include taxidermy chickens dressed in Edwardian-era formal wear, and a vast collection of first edition out-of-print art books and vintage modern furniture are also settled in among the sleek racks of high-end wares.

Maxfield is like a high-end, rock-'n'-roll museum carrying some of the most exquisite and eye-catching items for rockners who love designer pieces or anyone who appreciates modern luxury with a one-of-a-kind edge.

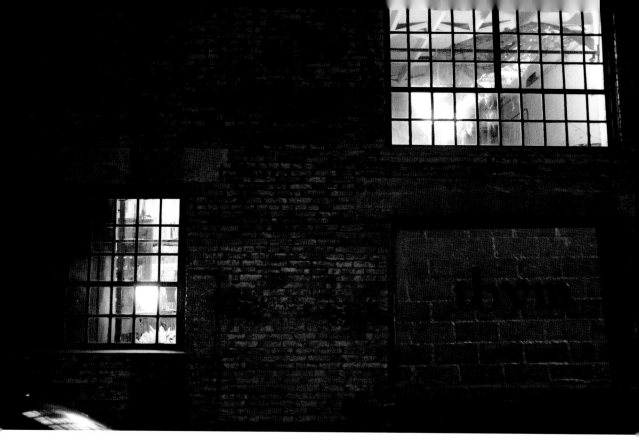

THVM
1317 Palmetto Street
Los Angeles, CA 90013
(213) 617-0667

Deep in downtown Los Angeles, nestled closer to the edge of the LA River than it is to any cookie-cutter strip mall, sits a store/studio and conceptual space called Thvm (pronounced them), housed in a hundred-year-old former paint factory that shows obvious signs of its age—but that's just the way owners and designers Olga Nazarova and Brian Kim like it.

The two clothing industry vets (she designed the rock-inspired, slightly avant-garde women's ready-to-wear line for Endovanera and he started the Work Custom denim label) launched their own denim collection, also called Thvm, and opened the retail space and studio not only to house their daily operations but also to further merchandise their line by filling the store with images and objects that continuously inspire them.

"We opened the Thvm store as a place to showcase our current denim and knit line. It's a place for our customers to come and see the inspiration behind the brand," says Nazarova, who along with Kim works with local artists to develop all-natural dyes for their jeans—often straight from the garden.

Thvm also carries like-minded designers such as Raquel Allegra, Cerre, and Arielle De Pinto, but it primarily stocks their sleek and skinny jeans for men and women. To add to the overall visual experience, Nazarova and Kim also produce a biannual publication called *Thvm Rag*—a magazine of sorts, filled with images that inspire and inform their line as well as artwork from local and global artists.

The art is not limited just to their publication. The interior of their brick store is curated with work from artists such as Ishi Glinsky and Caiti Hawkins, which provides another level of visual stimulation and at the same time enhances the gritty yet charming character of the structure.

It's a far cry from the all-white, sun-lit spaces of Rodeo Drive, but Thvm and other creative ventures like them that are also thriving in the artist-filled enclave of downtown LA have formed a community in the area where ideas flow between design, art, music, and fashion.

"Thvm is an acronym for 'This here very moment,'" says Nazarova. "The name seemed like a proper choice as we are more of a creative collective."

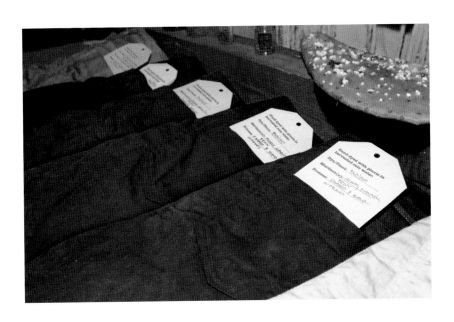

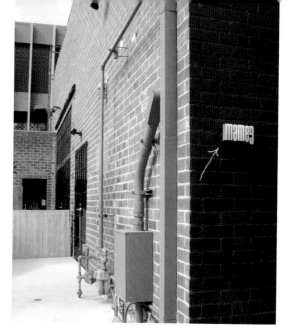

MAMEG

9970 S. Santa Monica Blvd.
Beverly Hills, CA 90212
(310) 826-4142

When it comes to destination shopping spots for the most intriguing and cleverly edited items in Los Angeles, people flock to an unassuming brick building settled in the back of a parking lot in Beverly Hills. Mameg is an airy, light-filled boutique that sits behind the Maison Martin Margiela store on Little Santa Monica Blvd. near the border of Beverly Hills and Century City.

Owner Sonia Eram initially opened her store in 1996 in Brentwood. In 2007 she moved into a 4,700-square-foot space that previously housed an auto repair shop, a golf store, and lastly a church and that she shares with Maison Martin Margiela's LA outpost. The two stores are connected by a gold-mirrored corridor inside and share a similar edgy, artsy, and avant-garde aesthetic.

Eram has a reputation for stocking beyond interesting and many times very hard-to-find items that she displays with the precision of a museum curator—but without the intimidation factor that comes with precious artifacts. Though many of the pieces are pricey, they are hung and shelved in a way one would carefully place them in their home, showcasing their beauty and specialness.

Lines like Cosmic Wonder, Hussein Chalayan, Bernhard Willhelm, Jil Sander, Viktor & Rolf, and Bless hang in limited quantity around the perimeter of the rectangular space. Anchoring the space in the center of the store are a large white couch and an eighteenth-century English partners desk at which Eram works as customers shop around her.

Anyone looking for a unique runway piece or just something completely off the mainstream radar is bound to find it here. Eram's sensibility for modern design with an edge shines through in every item she stocks.

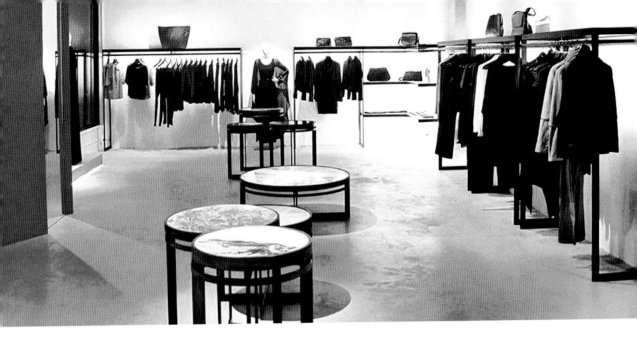

CERRE

8920 Melrose Ave.
West Hollywood, CA 90069
(310) 385-9051

Clayton and Flavie Webster, the husband-and-wife design duo behind the Cerre line have a penchant for luxurious leathers, sleek and simple lines, and a rocker-meets-effortlessly-chic attitude behind both their personal style and the look of their collection, which is housed in their modern and minimal-looking atelier in the heart of West Hollywood.

The former models met while working in Paris and developed a taste for the sumptuous and simple leathers many Parisian designers were manipulating into avant-garde items such as second-skin jackets and motorcycle-inspired pants. The two aim for balance between calm and chaos in their work with the stamp of traditional craftsmanship and a timeless and aspirational appeal. Their line, of course, also has a touch of rebellious rocker attitude and a cool, almost Goth sense of mystery.

The collection includes bags, jackets, hats, and pants made from buttery leathers, generally black, tan, or gray, often with fringe or an easy and interesting drape on the back of jackets, as well as solid cotton jersey separates, also done in a palette of earthy and versatile neutral tones.

The shop is undoubtedly a destination stop, and its musician, celebrity, and fashion-insider clientele have no trouble popping in to check out the latest leather items the store has to offer. To add to the tactile and handcrafted appeal, all samples are now sewn together in the back of the store on one of three sewing machines. It looks and feels like a high-end atelier doused with a shot of gritty, rocker edginess that captures both a time-honored tradition of leatherwork, plus an undeniable slouchy cool that makes sense on the stages of the world's most famous rock arenas as well as styled into easy, casual basics.

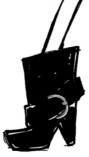

HOW TO GET THE LOOK
rocker

The rocker look is a tough-as-nails mix of black leather, edgy basics, and fierce accessories—all worn with a bold attitude and strong sense of confidence.

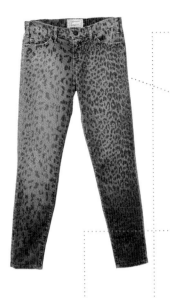

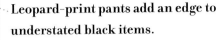

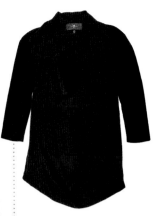

Leopard-print pants add an edge to understated black items.

Gunmetal gray nail lacquer works like a hard-hitting accessory.

Spikes and studs are a rocker must and can be worn on everything from bangles to evening bags.

A snakeskin bag brings a touch of the exotic and makes a luxe statement.

Killer black shoes are rocker staples. Try ankle boots for day and sexy cage heels for evening.

A twisted chain necklace adds texture and toughness.

Smudge on smoky black eyeliner to give any outfit a sultry finish.

Gold wire-frame sunglasses done in an edgy shape temper heavier, black basics.

A short, sexy dress with tough zipper details can be worn on its own or over leather leggings with a pair of high-heeled ankle booties.

A fitted black top with an interesting detail has a rocker edge even when worn with a pair of simple skinny jeans.

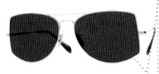

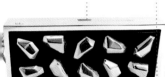

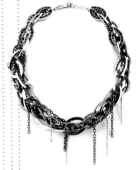

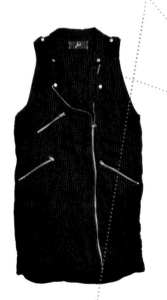

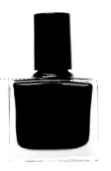

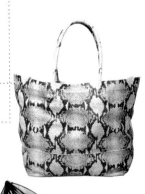

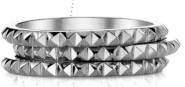

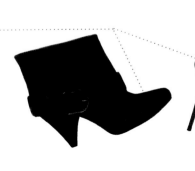

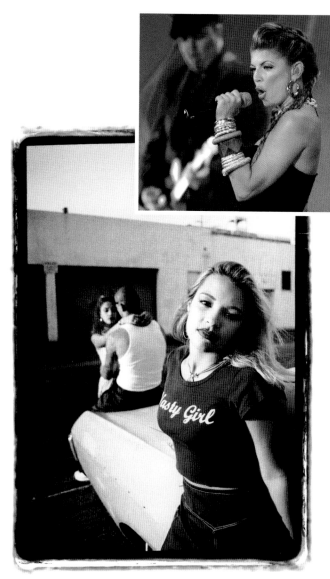

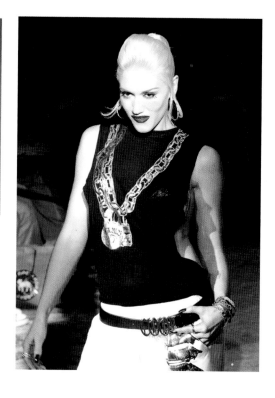

CLOCKWISE FROM TOP LEFT: **Fergie** of the Black Eyed Peas during the 2005 MuchMusic Video Awards in Toronto, Canada. **Gwen Stefani** during New York Fashion Week, spring 2006. **Kat Von D**, famous tattoo artist and star of *LA Ink*, signs copies of *The Tattoo Chronicles* at Barnes & Noble, October 30, 2010, in Florida. **Miley Cyrus** performs at the 2010 Annual MuchMusic Video Awards in Toronto, Canada. "La Sickass Angel Baby," 1996, Los Angeles, CA, photographed by Estevan Oriol.

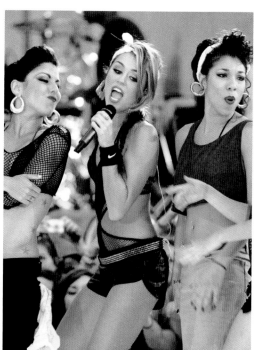

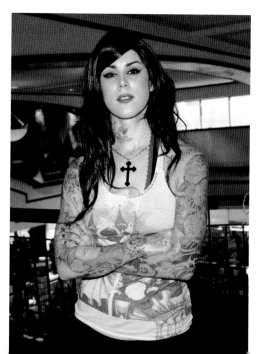

chola-style

When I moved to LA it was the late 70s but the cholas, the chicano gang girls, were still working a mid-60s look. In other words, they looked like Amy Winehouse. Genius! I think the style is always inspiring. Everybody has a little bad girl inside them who fantasizes about stashing a pointy comb in her beehive.

—SIMON DOONAN,
CREATIVE AMBASSADOR-
AT-LARGE FOR BARNEYS NEW YORK

There's no mistaking Southern California chola-style: the pin-thin eyebrows, meticulous turned-up flick of liquid eyeliner, and the tough but glamorous look that Gwen Stefani among others have spun into a million-dollar career, built in large part on "personal style."

This quintessentially California look has permeated pop culture over the past two decades, but its origins have deep cultural and political roots that started with the children of working-class Mexican immigrants and still binds many people to their heritage. LA is home to a huge Mexican immigrant population and the city has long felt its rich cultural influence. As with other immigrant groups, many second-generation Mexican American teenagers who grew up in the United States from the 1920s through the 1940s struggled not only to assimilate to adolescent life in a country still riddled with racism but also to maintain ties to their family's culture and live up to its expectations.

The inevitable search for a sense of self that followed led them on a search for social, cultural, and sartorial expression—and through that journey a subculture and a style were born.

The forces of Americanization were major factors in how this identity developed. Everything from the infectious sound of swing music to the glamorous film actresses of Hollywood influenced Mexican American kids who were living in Los Angeles during the first half of the twentieth century.

They articulated their look and attitude by fusing their two worlds together, trying to navigate between adopting the norms of a predominantly white society and expressing pride in their Mexican roots.

The creation of this subculture within the Mexican American community started in the 1920s when women began emulating the look of flappers. Their identity started to solidify as strong and somewhat rebellious during the 1940s when zoot suits were criminalized and Mexican Americans who wore them became the target of cops.

As the Chicano movement swept through America in the 1960s, a sense of liberation and pride arose within the community and Mexican American artists, writers, and activists were prolific and effective in giving minorities a voice.

Still, the search for a collective identity continued, and style elements from the 1940s remained a part of how many Mexican American women looked and dressed—a nod not only to a pivotal time in their history but also to a glamorous and highly stylized aesthetic.

The evolution of this woman by the 1960s became known as a chola (a feminine version of the word cholo, which was historically used as an ethnic slur referring to people of mixed American Indian heritage). The word has taken on multiple connotations over the years and during the 1960s was adopted as a term used to describe the look and affiliation with a gang (though that was certainly not always the case). Today we use the term "chola" when talking about the clothing and distinctive makeup style indicative of this community—not necessarily in reference to gangs.

The chola look is definitive, and started to gel into the tough, boy-meets-girl look we know it to be today during the 1970s. The style, which denotes ethnic unity and a streetwise breed of glamour, still influences everyone from style watchers and pop stars to designers and makeup artists.

Pencil-thin eyebrows drawn with Sharpie-like precision are one of the style's most recognizable elements, but there are also the multiple layers of mascara and vinyl-black liquid eyeliner ending in a pointed, upturned flick. These details served as inspiration for celebrities including Gwen Stefani, Fergie, and tattoo artist and reality TV star Kat Von D.

Thin, arched eyebrows are associated with the chola look, but it's a beauty ritual with a history dating back to the flappers of the 1920s, a time when immigration from Mexico was at a high due to the abundance of work available during and soon after World War I.

Mexican American women during the early 20s began absorbing many of the American fashion influences that were swirling around them and flappers embodied the sense of freedom and rebelliousness they craved. They began emulating flapper-style, such as bobbed hair and drop-waist dresses.

These young women, eager to find their own identity, were drawn to American movies, music, and dance and used the pop culture of the 1920s and 30s to hone their style.

Soon there were chicano flappers, who began to cut their hair in bobs, dying their raven locks red and wearing the same style of makeup as the caucasian flappers. A song written at the time called "Las Pelonas" or "the bobbed heads" refers to all of the dyed red and bobbed hair on Mexican American women in the 20s.

Just as flappers were seen as rebellious at that time, the Mexican American women who emulated the look also created some scandal within their community, because they were going against the traditional and deeply Catholic heritage they came from. The struggle of Mexican American women for identity in American culture had officially started, and by the 1940s it would not only encompass a whole lifestyle and attitude, but it would also set the stage for the look of the cholas and homegirls.

In the 1940s, a more organized sense of identity and style emerged within LA's Mexican American community and many of the young men and women were known as pachucos (men) and pachucas (women)—a term for teenagers and young adults who dressed more outrageously than their peers and frequented dance halls for the upbeat music and swing dancing.

One of the strongest images associated with the pachuco subculture was its signature ensemble, consisting of a long pinstripe jacket and baggy tapered pants, often worn with a fedora and wallet chain. Known as the zoot suit, it was a hallmark of 1940s fashion that the pachucos picked up from African American performers like Cab Calloway.

KAT VON D

I am constantly inspired by my surroundings—I think I was just lucky enough to have been brought up in Los Angeles—a place where the mixtures of cultures and subcultures not only influence my approach to my art, but my personal look as well.

Along with their zoot suits, pachucos sported pompadours and slick ducktails that pointed down toward the nape of their neck.

The women, pachucas, wore letterman-style sweaters, draped slacks, or a full, knee-length skirt, high bobby socks, and huaraches or "zombie shoes" as they were sometimes referred to.

Their makeup was not unlike the Hollywood starlets of the time who were under the influence of movie studios and makeup artists like Max Factor. Their eyebrows were plucked pencil thin and their lips were painted a dramatic deep red. The pachucas also rolled their hair into a pompadouresque-style by inserting a hair tool called a "rat" in order to gain height and a smooth rolled-back coif that was like an exaggerated version of the victory rolls popular during the 1940s.

Some speculate that pachucas hid weapons in their victory rolls and pompadours and the higher the hairdo the more likely she might be concealing a weapon. While the idea has all the makings of a cool Hollywood subplot, it's more likely urban legend than reality.

The pachucos and pachucas were not all gang members, but outsiders saw the subculture as often dangerous and at the very least, rebellious. Many who sported the style were simply following a fashion trend, not unlike recent music subcultures like rockabilly or punk. But by 1943 it didn't seem to matter, and because of an incident known as the Sleepy Lagoon murder the pachuco/pachuca look began to be seen as violent and criminal.

The Sleepy Lagoon incident involved the murder of a Mexican American man at a reservoir in southeast Los Angeles for which a group of young pachucos were charged and put on trial. Their zoot suits—well known as a part of this subculture—were instantly seen by police as defiant and rebellious. Suddenly this style of dress, as well as anyone who dared to continue wearing it, became a provocation for police attention or incarceration.

The Sleepy Lagoon murder sparked a chaotic string of sometimes-violent protests that started in Los Angeles but spread throughout other major U.S. cities. They were called the Zoot Suit Riots, which made wearing a zoot suit a symbol of rebellion and antipatriotism. Zoot suits were further criminalized by the media and law enforcement as a sign of gang affiliation and violence. Today zoot suits are still worn for their significance in Mexican American history as a sign of confidence and a symbol of overcoming conflict.

The look of the pachucos and pachucas and the subculture created during the 1940s have become a sartorial expression of chicano pride and history for the Mexican American community, especially in Los Angeles. And elements of the pachuco/pachuca looks, such as the fedora, high-waist pants, suspenders, pencil-thin eyebrows, and dark lipstick, carried through to the 1960s and 70s when pachucas became known as cholas.

The cholas, like the pachucas, riffed on popular American styles but added an edgy spin that helped define the look. Mexican American women worked elements into their clothing and makeup that expressed a tougher and more self-assured attitude as female gangs became more organized.

Chola-style was a variation on the look of the pachucas. They wore short skirts, cat-eye makeup, and intense, dark plum-colored lipstick, a beauty detail that would become a mainstay of the chola look.

Cholas also still had those thin, arched eyebrows, but the hairstyle changed slightly from the pachucas' 40s pompadour (which was teased on top but long and straight toward the bottom) to the still somewhat large and feathered hair popular during the 1970s. The high hair, eye makeup, and severe lipstick was a definite mix of hard and soft, similar to the strong, glamorous, and confident look of the pachucas.

Film director Allison Anders—who directed arguably the most realistic on-screen description of 1990s homegirl culture in Echo Park, *Mi Vida Loca*—moved to LA's San Fernando Valley in 1969 and became immersed in the lowrider and chola scene that was emerging from the Latino culture in the area. She recalls a slight punk influence that emerged among cholas in Los Angeles during the 1970s, which seemed to go both ways (punks influencing the cholas and the cholas inspiring the punks). She specifically cites the black rubber bands (that were actually a part taken from the engine of a car) that cholas wore as bracelets. "They got elaborate with them and would attach them to a finger and it looked very spiderwebby," says Anders. "The cholas started it and it totally makes sense because it came from a car."

By the mid-1970s cholas had abandoned the skirts more common to the style of the pachucas, and a more masculine look started to emerge and coalesce with their community-specific makeup and signature hair. The women began to band together and assert their own sense of toughness and strength. Skirts were a thing of the past and replaced with baggy pants not unlike the ones the men wore.

Their new look was quite literally boy meets girl, with cholas adopting both masculine and feminine elements, taking on a tough side while still staying true to the traditionally feminine role of women within the Mexican culture. They took the feminine aspect and the typical male role and put an exaggerated spin on both to create a look that was finally their own.

By the 1990s cholas were referred to as homegirls, yet the signature aspects of chola-style remained. The thin eyebrows and distinct cat eyeliner were consistent with cholas—as was the pouf of hair, which was created by teasing up their bangs and pulling half of the hair up or all of it totally back into a ponytail.

But homegirls also began to incorporate slightly more severe aspects into their makeup by donning white eye shadow, a stark contrast to the jet-black eyeliner and mascara. The dark plum and red lipstick worn by cholas during the 1970s and 80s morphed into brown or very dark lip liner surrounding light brown or otherwise totally nude lips. Accessories included bandannas, gold hoop earrings, and athletic shoes like Nike Cortez—not unlike what their male counterparts (or homeboys) wore.

Anders's film *Mi Vida Loca* captures the general look of homegirls in LA during the 1990s with the main characters—all based on women she encountered while living in the neighborhood for eight years—outfitted in chinos, baggy jeans, and athletic or oversize T-shirts.

"There was still some shaving of the eyebrows, tail eyeliner, white around the eyes, dark eyeliner, and nude lips," says Anders. "They were not trying to look pretty. They were fierce. It was like armor in order to not be so vulnerable."

The blend of masculine and feminine brought about not only a look that was sexy and strong, but it also gave women who wore it a sense of confidence, power, and identity.

Alice Armendariz (a.k.a. Alice Bag), former lead singer of LA punk band the Bags, grew up in East LA and was influenced by chola-style. "I adopted the dramatic use of eyeliner that made cholas look fierce, before fierce was a fashionista term," she says. "There was a lack of innocence or pretense in their dress. Chola-style was unapologetically sexy and female, assertive and confident, yet so far out of the mainstream that no one dared call it pretty. I absorbed some of that style and brought it with me to punk."

The idea of being tough while still maintaining a strong sense of femininity has been a solid source of inspiration for girls who have grown up around the subculture, as well as pop stars, singers, and celebrities who find the glamorous-but-tough vibe appealing and aesthetically on point with conveying confidence and a sense of mystery.

Gwen Stefani has cited the chola look many times as a major influence in her style and references key elements in her L.A.M.B clothing line. When she launched her line in 2005, she said she admired the chola look for the "contrast between being overly girlie, with long red nails and masses of makeup, and being masculine and tough."

The aesthetic has been an obvious influence on Stefani's personal style in the form of pompadours anchored by long slick ponytails, long oval-shaped red fingernails, large belt buckles with old English script, brick-red lipstick, bandannas, and overly baggy pants worn with "wife beater" tank tops.

The chola and homegirl look has also influenced pop star Fergie, who, like Stefani, is from Southern California. In the video for her 2006 song "London Bridge," the singer sports pin-thin eyebrows (a feature she had for several years with the Black Eyed Peas) a cutoff white tank top, and plaid, menswear-inspired knee-length shorts.

Tattoo artist and reality TV star Kat Von D includes two shades of lipstick in her makeup line that reference the chola culture. One is a deep dark purple called "Homegirl" and the other a pale, barely there nude called "Mi Vida Loca." Her personal style is also influenced by the look, evidenced by her cat-eye makeup, heavily lined lips, and smattering of colorful and ornate tattoos.

"Los Angeles is a place where the mix of culture and subcultures not only influence my approach to my art, but my personal look as well," says Von D. "Everything from the architecture of downtown, to the murals painted in alleyways and on lowriders, to the prominent Mexican culture all play a huge role in who I am."

From pop stars to suburban girls experimenting with style, the chola look originally represented the street-tough aesthetic of gang-affiliated females, but it has since permeated mainstream and pop culture for the mix of power, glamour, and femininity that started in the shadows of male counterparts but emerged on its own as a symbol of strength.

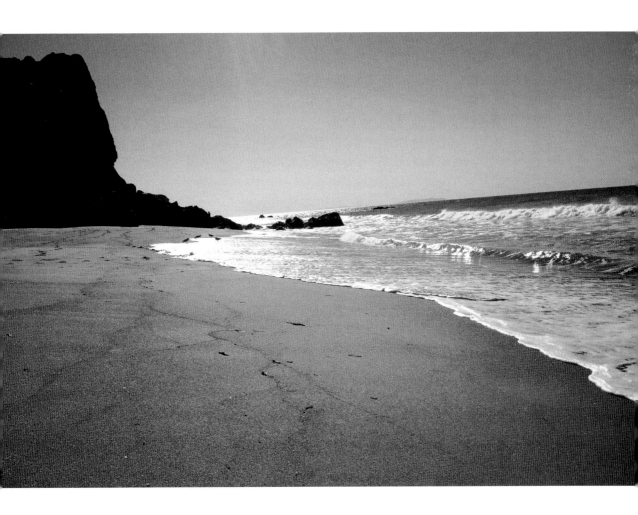

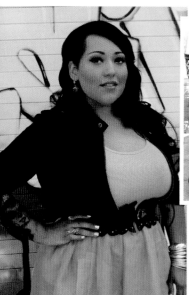
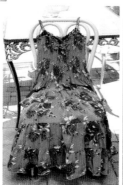
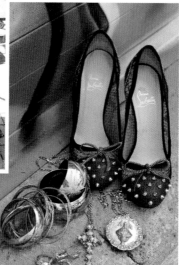
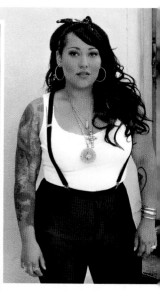

Name: **DALINA REBOLLO** Hometown: EAST LA AND HIGHLAND PARK, CA

Occupation: HAIRSTYLIST

How would you describe your style?
My style is adventurous and approachable chola. I guess that means I look tough, but dress cute and have my friends' backs. Being a Mexican American I try to show my culture through my style. I wear a lot of Virgin Mary jewelry and Day of the Dead–inspired prints and large vibrant florals.

Who are your style icons?
Style icons include Lady Gaga, Gwen Stefani, JLo, and Selena. All these women have their own style and are true badasses.

What are your go-to pieces and/or your favorite item in your closet? And what would you consider a signature aspect of your style?
My go-to pieces include wild-patterned leggings. I also love rompers and onesies and anything that has crazy prints or patterns on it. I like platform shoes. They're comfortable to work in all day and make my short legs look longer.

What is the last thing you bought and what is your must-have piece of clothing right now?
The last thing bought is this crazy green Betsey Johnson summer dress with multicolored roses all over it. My must-have piece of clothing is my black romper with a bustle. I make it more Mexi by wearing it with a wife beater and crazy gold jewelry.

Name some other things you feel distinguish your style.
I wear at least one piece of my grandmother's jewelry. She passed away when I was twelve. I remember her as a very fancy and glamorous woman. I inherited every piece of jewelry she left behind. I have tons of Jesus chains, Virgin Marys, gold coins, hoops, and bangles. Another accessory I cannot leave behind is my tattoos. I have a sleeve on my right arm that is indicative of my culture.

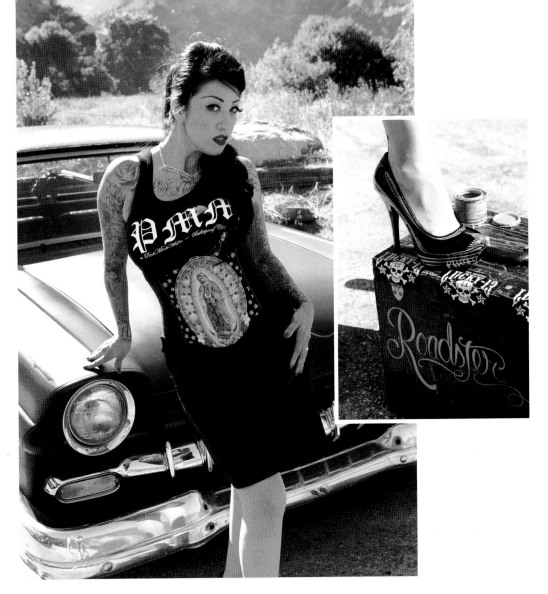

Name: **LATINA VAMP** (a.k.a. LV)   Hometown: AZUSA, CA
Occupation: CEO AND FOUNDER OF A CLOTHING COMPANY

How would you describe your style?
I describe my style as "rock-a-chola."

Who are your style icons?
People who have inspired my style in the past are women I grew up watching in early Latin cinema like Maria Felix and Dolores del Rio.

What are your go-to pieces in your closet?
You will most likely catch me wearing either my chola belt with my initial, my studded belt with skull buckle, or my corset—and always in heels.

What is the last thing you bought?
The last thing I bought was a tattoo drawing of two traditional-style black panthers dressed like cholos fighting each other.

What are a few things you feel distinguish your style?
My long black hair and tattoos. I'm pretty easy to spot because I'm the only one with PinkMinkMafia tattooed on her chest. I also love wearing a flower in my hair. It keeps me feeling girly.

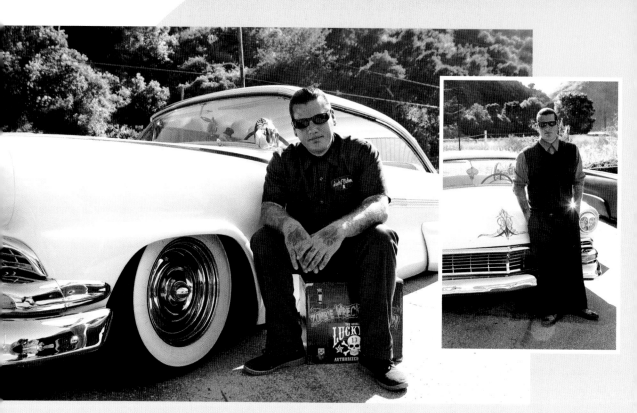

Name: RICKY ROADSTER Hometown: LOS ANGELES, CA
Occupation: CUSTOM CAR PAINTER, SHOP OWNER, AND BARBER

How would you describe your style?
Classy, ol' school, 1950s Kustom Kar Kulture of LA.

Do you have any style icons?
Musicians and gangsters from the 1930s through the 1960s including John Dillinger, Billy Lee Riley, Joe Clay, the Midnighters, and the Flamingos.

What are your favorite items in your closet?
My Zombie Wrecking Crew vest, brown-and-tan wool clicker coat, and Lucky 13 button-ups.

What would you consider a signature aspect of your style?
My slicked-back hair, my tattoos, my paint box, pinstripe sunglasses, hats, and winos.

What is the last thing you bought?
Mack Blue Wrap pinstriping brush and pack of Marlboro Reds.

Who are your favorite designers? And what are your go-to places to shop?
Lucky 13, World Famous Hawleywood's Barbershop, Costa Mesa.

What are your grooming habits?
Shower, straight razor shave, No. 9 Aftershave, Layrite Pomade.

Do you have a signature scent?
Old Spice and paint.

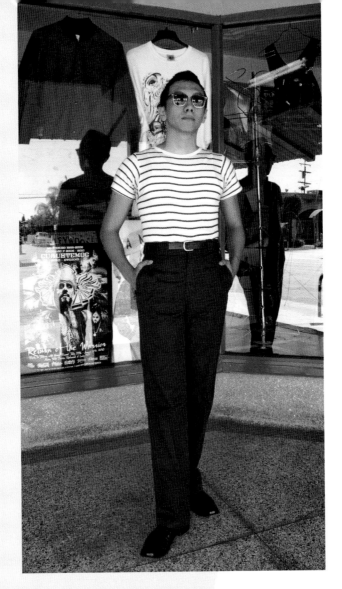

Name: GUILLERMO CUEVAS

Hometown: SOUTH GATE, CA   Occupation: STUDENT

How would you describe your style?
My style is classic and I don't stick to one certain time period.

What are your favorite items in your closet?
My vintage slacks are my favorite thing in my closet and my Pendleton shirts being a close second.

What is the last thing you bought?
The last thing I bought is a custom-made wool letterman cardigan for my school.

What are your grooming habits? Do you have a signature scent?
I get a haircut once a month, which is when my hair gets uncontrollably messy. Signature scent would have to be the vanilla scented pomade in my hair.

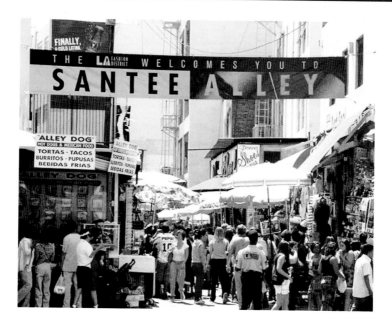

SANTEE ALLEY

Two blocks between Santee St., Maple Ave.,
Olympic Blvd., and Twelfth St.

Santee Alley is the two-block stretch in the heart of downtown LA's Fashion District, where vendors carrying everything from straw fedoras to knockoff designer bags gather each day to sell their wares to the masses of shoppers looking for good deals on a vast array of merchandise. The Alley has been home to vendors since the 1970s, when they began selling their overrun of clothing out of the back of their stores and into the alley. Today it's consistently packed with anyone looking for accessories, trendy clothes, and interested in immersing themselves in a multicultural outdoor excursion that feels quintessentially LA.

The setting is a sensory overload in the best way possible, with clothing, bags, shoes, and jewelry displayed on tables and shelves throughout the alley. Besides the heaps of things to buy, there is a festival-style atmosphere that includes music blaring from a nearby boom box, bubbles wafting out of stalls from an automatic machine, churro carts, and other street food vendors—all of which make the trip to the Alley an exciting and totally unique experience.

The 150 stalls at Santee Alley tend to carry a lot of the same thing. Whatever the hot trend is at the time—whether it's jeggings, bedazzled T-shirts, gladiator sandals, or baggy jeans—they're bound to have it in abundance. Prices are low and there's generally room to bargain with vendors at the pedestrian-only marketplace situated between Maple and Santee Streets that runs from Olympic to Pico Boulevards.

And though merchandise might change

with mass fashion trends, there are some items that remain constant. The walkways are peppered with inexpensive gems like Converse sneakers, socks, sunglasses, bootleg CDs and DVDs, packs of white T-shirts, white tank tops, and kiosks selling all kinds of gold jewelry like twisted hoops, cross pendants, sets of dainty bangles, and large and customizable belt buckles.

It's a far cry from the bank-breaking high heels at the department stores near Rodeo Drive, but the atmosphere as well as the loads of affordable merchandise are worth a trip down to the Alley whether you're in the market to score a good deal on some gold jewelry or just interested in having an eye-opening and exciting out-door shopping experience.

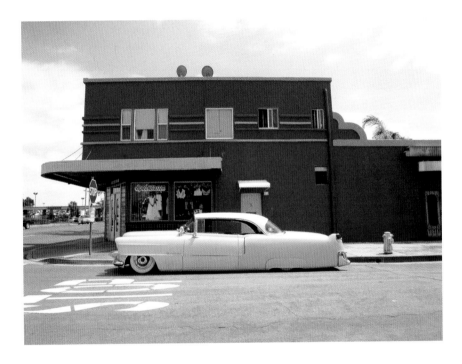

EL PACHUCO
801 S. Harbor Blvd.
Fullerton, CA 92832
(714) 526-3743

LA resident and former jewelry retailer Phyllis Estrella first became familiar with the cultural significance and 1940s aes-thetic of a pachuco when in 1978 she saw the play *El Pachuco*, starring Edward James Olmos. Olmos's character, also called El Pachuco, appealed to Estrella, who was struck by the confident demeanor and sharp and colorful zoot suit he wore as well as the historical link that the suit and the men who wore them conveyed.

Estrella began her zoot suit business, named El Pachuco after the play, Olmos's character, and the Mexican American pachuco culture that formed during the 1940s, first by selling just the long wallet chains commonly swinging from the pockets of zoot suit pants. She eventually found a tailor in Southern California who was skilled at making the suits and production quickly began on creating a line of authentic zoot suits that initially appealed mainly to the Mexican population in Southern California and eventually started attracting attention from people all over the world who appreciated the retro look and instant swagger of the suits.

The store, located in Fullerton, California, houses the El Pachuco line of suits, along with accessories like fedoras, wing-tip shoes, and wallet chains. In 2007, Estrella's daughter-in-law, Vanessa, started a women's counterpart to the El Pachuco line accurately named La Pachuca. She designs retro-inspired clothing that takes from the 1930s, 40s, and 50s, mixing high-waist sailor-style pants and body-conscious pencil skirts with full and flirty 50s-style dresses and ultrafeminine flowered headbands with silk-screened tank tops and T-shirts featuring work from artist Julian Mendoza who's known for his illustrations of pachucas.

"This look has never really gone away," says Vanessa Estrella. "It's a way for people to express themselves just like any other style. The [pachuco and pachuca look] has been passed down from generation to gen-eration. People's mothers used to dress like that, or their dads are pachucos. It all influences us today."

The 2000-square-foot store with a teal-and-pink 50s exterior carries not just ready-made zoot suits and all the accoutrement one might need to go along with them, but it also does a steady custom-made business for people who want a specific style, color, or stripe.

"The thing with our style is that we don't follow the latest trends," says Vanessa Estrella. "We stick to a certain era and the glamour of that era is really all we do. I think that's what the Latino community loves about it, that we are sticking to an era of clothing that is not found in just any store in the mall." The store has a strong presence in the city, advertising at rockabilly and lowrider car shows, both of which have a strong Latino following. But the unique look of El Pachuco and La Pachuca has had a global reach as the retro-style has permeated different cultures and countries. "We get customers from all over—Sweden, England, China, Japan—that all love this era," says Estrella. Between the ultraglamorous appeal of both the men's and women's collections and the deep-rooted heritage of the brand, it's not hard to see why.

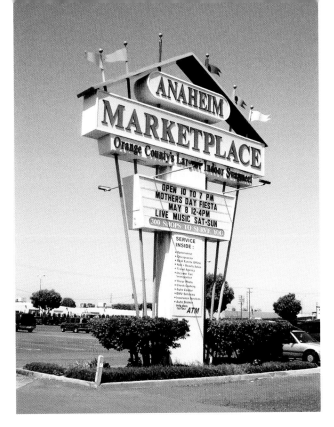

ANAHEIM INDOOR MARKETPLACE

1440 S. Anaheim Blvd.
Anaheim, CA 92805
(714) 999-0888

Anaheim may famously be home to the Magic Kingdom, but in the same city sits a 130,000-square-foot indoor marketplace housing over two hundred vendors selling everything from candy and car parts to *quinceañera* jewelry. Since 1991, the Anaheim Indoor Marketplace has been a one-stop shop, gathering place for the local community, live music venue, and source of vast culinary offerings, ranging from common comfort foods to the exotic.

In addition to the vendors selling T-shirts and work boots, there are massage therapists, optometrists, beauty salons, piercing and tattoo parlors, pet shops, fortune tellers, auto registration, a shoe repair, a 99-cent store, a check-cashing center, a piñata store, and a place to buy traditional Mexican folkloric clothing.

The lively ambiance blends a comprehensive shopping experience with food and music from traditional Latino culture, drawing visitors every weekend who shop, come to listen to live mariachi music, and eat from the massive food court, which has traditional Mexican fare like popular pork skin appetizers *tostilocos* and Tejuino, a drink originating from Guadalajara, Mexico.

The clothing and jewelry offerings are hard to miss, as stalls are filled with gold jewelry like crosses, medallions with saints, Mayan calendar pendants, sports team insignias, wheel-rim pendants, name-plate pendants, chunky thick hoop earrings, and ID bracelets. Clothing ranges from the utilitarian, including Dickies sweatshirts and slacks, to more colorful baseball caps and T-shirts ready for custom airbrushing, hoodies and hats emblazoned with "Los Angeles" on them, and perhaps most uniquely, T-shirts with a chola-style Marilyn Monroe on the front with the word "SoCal" written just beneath her high heels.

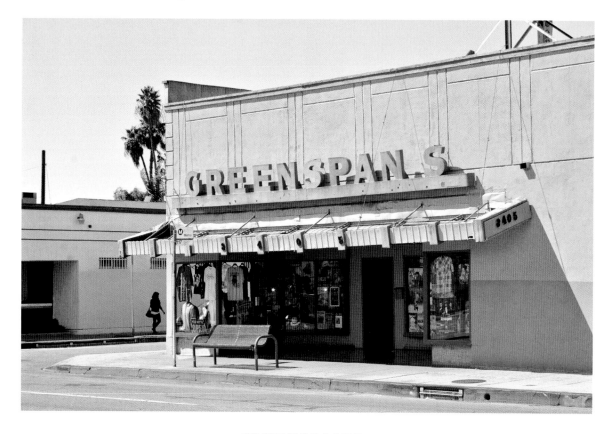

GREENSPAN'S
3405 Tweedy Blvd.
South Gate, CA 90280
(323) 566-5124

Greenspan's is the oldest family-owned lifestyle store west of Texas, and it's known for selling classic LA street-wear basics that attract everyone from Cypress Hill to NWA to Lady Gaga.

Situated in an unassuming gray building a few miles southeast of downtown LA, the 6,500-square-foot space is filled with vintage zoot suits, fedoras, wino shoes, tie bars, vintage Levi's, and a robust quantity of Pendleton button-down shirts. Each piece is a nod to classic 1940s and 50s style and appeals to people who still appreciate the traditional pachuco look.

What started as a junior department store in Watts in 1928 has evolved into a men's emporium of original and covetable pieces that reflect an old-school LA look.

There is a distinctly 1940s and 50s vibe and unmistakably West Coast aesthetic to every item. The Greenspan family doesn't just sell it; they live it.

On any given day, Evan Greenspan—with the help of his son and daughter—can be found manning the register in his button-down Pendleton, carpenter-style jeans, and classic Hush Puppies.

Items like winos, Hush Puppies loafers, Pendletons, zoot suits, and fedoras all carry the history of LA's surfer and cholo subculture from back in the 1960s and 70s. And the people who still rock the old-school look come to Greenspan's for the one-stop shopping experience and mix of dead stock, vintage, and authentically Southern California pieces.

Greenspan's has even taken to reproducing items that some companies stopped making to fill the demand, including their own style of wool varsity jacket, classic pea coats, carpenter jeans, and fedoras.

The store isn't just a favorite of celebrities like Snoop Dogg and Ryan Gosling. It also appeals to designers for labels ranging from RRL to O'Neill, who scour the expanse of merchandise for the rich history, heritage, and solid inspiration that comes from the classics.

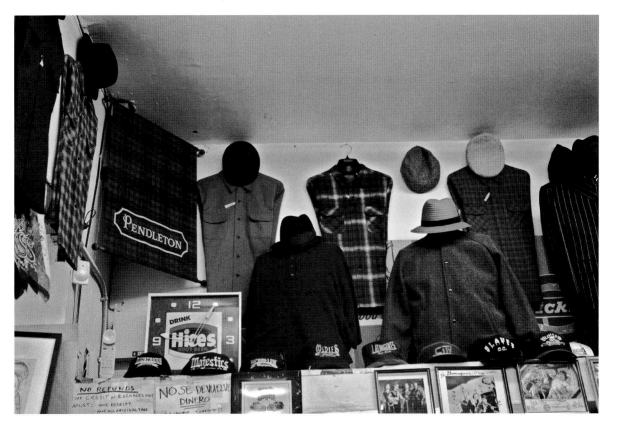

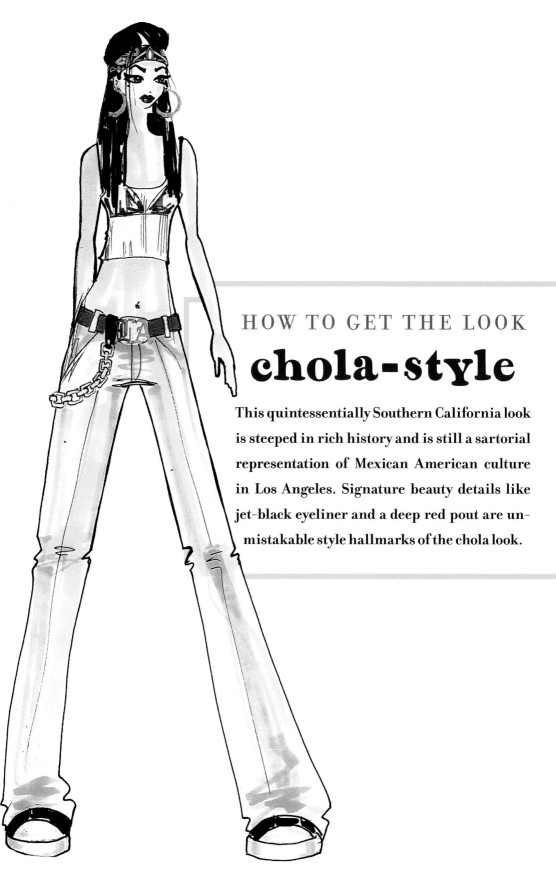

chola-style

This quintessentially Southern California look is steeped in rich history and is still a sartorial representation of Mexican American culture in Los Angeles. Signature beauty details like jet-black eyeliner and a deep red pout are unmistakable style hallmarks of the chola look.

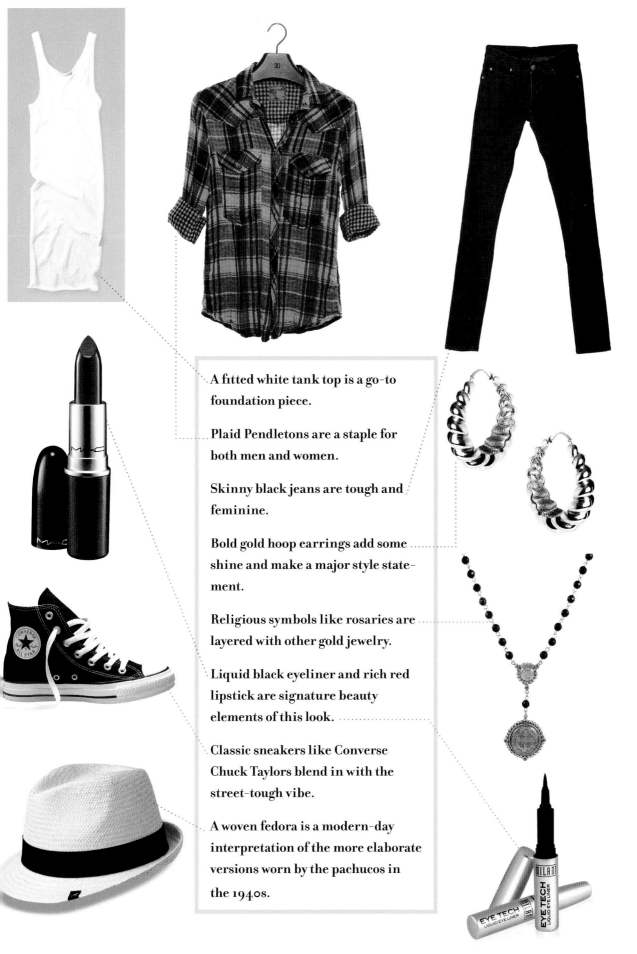

A fitted white tank top is a go-to foundation piece.

Plaid Pendletons are a staple for both men and women.

Skinny black jeans are tough and feminine.

Bold gold hoop earrings add some shine and make a major style statement.

Religious symbols like rosaries are layered with other gold jewelry.

Liquid black eyeliner and rich red lipstick are signature beauty elements of this look.

Classic sneakers like Converse Chuck Taylors blend in with the street-tough vibe.

A woven fedora is a modern-day interpretation of the more elaborate versions worn by the pachucos in the 1940s.

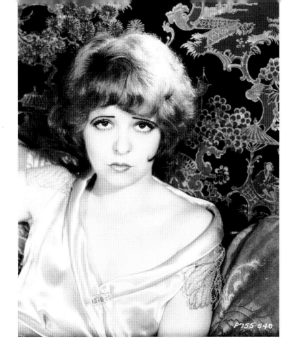

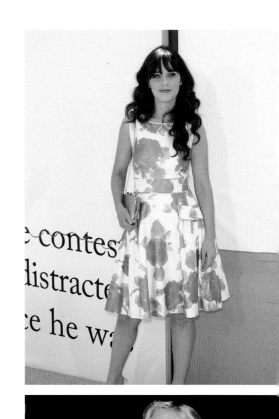

Clockwise from top left: ca. 1929: A melancholy **Clara Bow** (1905–65) in a satin dress. July 10, 2011: Actress **Zooey Deschanel** attends the premiere of Disney's *Winnie the Pooh* at Walt Disney Studios in Burbank, CA. November 13, 2010: Actress **Kirsten Dunst** arrives at MOCA Presents: Envisioned by Artist Doug Aitken at MOCA, Grand Avenue in Los Angeles, CA. Ca. 1950: American actress **Lucille Ball** (1911–89) with her husband, **Desi Arnaz** (1917–86). July 4, 2009: **Jenny Lewis** poses backstage after her performance at the River to River Festival at Battery Park in New York City, NY.

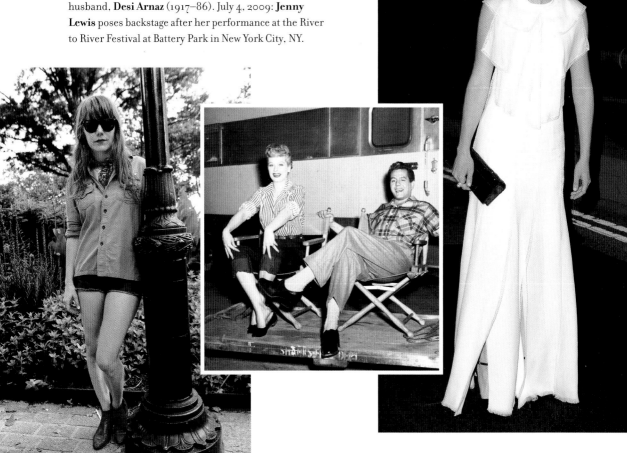

indie eclectic

More than any place I can think of, LA is a true collage-city: desert, ocean, mountains, hills, urban-centers, and suburban flats-and the style is by nature varied, complex, camera ready, and yes, incredibly relevant and influential.

— CHINA CHOW

Vintage pieces are at the core of most contemporary trends, acting as a reference point to anchor key styles from decades past. And Los Angeles boasts an abundant supply of some of the best retro pieces because of its temperate climate, which prevents fabrics from aging too rapidly, and vintage-hungry Southern California shoppers, who are inspired by the city's creative and eclectic music and art scenes. That's why the indie eclectic look—a style comprised of vintage or vintage-inspired items worn with a contemporary flair—flourishes in LA.

The men and women who embody an eclectic and more independent attitude toward life, style, music, and art thrive in the hilly neighborhoods and eastside enclaves of Silverlake, Los Feliz, and Echo Park, which are filled with artisanal coffee shops, small records stores, and gritty music venues. They tend to cite more literary and cinematic references—creating looks that combine unusual elements and are often steeped in history—when it comes to getting dressed. There is a maverick sensibility to the style and often a story or strong reference behind every ensemble, blending thrift store treasures with book worm and tomboy staples, as well as up-and-coming designers, for a look that's unexpected and never, ever cookie-cutter.

There is always something personal (from heirloom jewelry or a boyfriend's old blazer), irreverent, and often askew about their clothes. Girls have a doll-like appeal, favoring kicky vintage dresses and flat oxfords or loafers; they are sentimental and generally look more sweetheart than sex kitten.

Actress Zooey Deschanel flawlessly embodies the indie eclectic girl, with her retro-fueled wardrobe, musical talent, and an offbeat sense of humor that has endearingly earned her the title of "adorkable." She, like many other indie eclectic individuals, favors 50s- and 60s-style dresses with a knee-length, pleated skirt or tiered ruffles and a blouse featuring details like a Peter Pan collar or 40s-style nautical flourishes. There is a clear nod to the past in everything she wears, whether it's a strapless gown with a grosgrain ribbon sash worn to an awards show or wide-leg jeans and a preppy, checked blazer for a more buttoned-up look. The silhouette is always antiquated, which seems to suit her body type and personality perfectly.

This blend of humor, awkwardness, and adorableness is the antithesis of the airbrushed reality-show stars and overtanned celebrities who have been so ubiquitous in pop culture, making it a refreshing departure from the artificial and seemingly impossible to attain. There is a charm to the look that is enticing, and though the polished and tailored pieces of the past are at the core of this style, it is still worn with a nonchalant, Southern California ease. It's almost along the lines of theme dressing, but in a good way, taking an era and diluting the style down so it isn't too literal and makes sense to modern times. It's flea market chic, but with a refined edge and air of whimsy, and people like Deschanel, Kirsten Dunst, and musicians Jenny Lewis and Karen O pull off this balance whether on stage, screen, or in their everyday lives.

These girls echo the same quirky and progressive attitude as the artistic and influential women who once lived in LA and helped shape the cultural and sartorial landscape of the city. From rebellious flappers and madcap TV stars to brooding beatniks, LA's indie attitude still thrives today in a way that blends a thrift store aesthetic with a thoroughly modern attitude.

Like the women of the past who broke boundaries in entertainment and society in LA, these individuals take normal ideals of establishment to make it better: They make it their own. They're voyeurs of everything going on around them, politically and culturally, basing their style on bits of pop culture—past and present—and tying it all together with intelligence, humor, wit, and whimsy.

Vintage clothing provides a strong wardrobe foundation for the indie girl and with the robust selection of vintage wares in Southern California, this style has often bucked trends and provided an alternative that is expressive, personal, and features a nod to zanier moments in the past. The mix of vintage with present-day pieces also represents an anti-mall look and a refusal of the generic norm.

LA vintage also inspires major designers and stylists, who come to town to snap up influential pieces that many times inform their collections. Doris Raymond, who, in addition to having an impressively stocked vintage retail store called The Way We Wore, keeps massive archives of vintage pieces for designers to reference. "The late great Alexander McQueen, Donatella Versace, Michael Kors, Donna Karan, Ralph Lauren, Spain's Loewe, Pucci, and Australia's Yeojin Bae have all come for inspiration," she says.

The Rose Bowl Flea Market also continues to be a huge resource for various designers, including denim-industry giants and celebs-turned-accessory designers-like Kate Bosworth. Bosworth and her stylist and design partner Cher Coulter frequent the Rose Bowl for vintage knickknacks and pieces that speak to their aesthetic and help to inform their jewelry line, JewelMint.

The flea market is a treasure trove of clothing, furniture, and objects from eras past just waiting to be discovered—as long as you have the time, the patience, and a keen eye for spotting gems.

Ironically, even mass-market brands understand the hunger for antiquated style and create lines that just look old. Anthropologie, Madewell, Urban Outfitters, and the rise of modcloth.com are examples of the turn to a more charming aesthetic. In LA, the style is accessorized with details like nerdy eyeglasses and face-framing bangs, but it's primarily the attitude and spirit, the marching-to-beat-of-their-own-drum approach to a look and lifestyle that sets the indie look apart.

The first half of the twentieth century in LA saw fierce women who were ahead of their time—raising eyebrows and challenging norms of society, sexuality, and style.

A brazen attitude, a signature look, and a vision to reconfigure their existing landscape are things flappers embodied, pushing societal boundaries with their clothing, hair, and rebellious natures.

The flappers represented a free spiritedness during the 1920s that emerged after World War I. They shed constricting corsets, long hair, and the reserved demeanor that were previously the social norm. The style, with its elaborately beaded drop-waist dresses, bobbed hair, and long cigarette holders provides a perfect mix of stylish glamour and a spirited bucking of the conventional notions about women and femininity.

Flappers were not necessarily unique to Los Angeles, as they were ubiquitous throughout the 1920s, but it was in LA specifically that women who embodied the flapper look appeared in films and perpetuated the look, style, and characteristics common to being a flapper. Women like Olive Thomas, Clara Bow, and Colleen Moore famously portrayed flappers onscreen and projected the idea of the modern woman.

Indie girls of today have adopted the beauty and clothing inspiration in their own look, sometimes incorporating it more extremely with a drop-waist cocktail frock on the red carpet, or more subtly with layered long necklaces or the heavy, blunt bangs commonly associated with a Louise Brooks—style bob.

On the street, everyday Indie girls dilute the style in a more casual and wearable manner, cutting their hair to their chin and pairing flat oxfords or loafers with both dresses and jeans. There's a tomboyish and rebellious nature to the style that has direct parallels to flappers of the 1920s.

Sartorial staples of an indie girl also include cute Peter Pan collars on a button-down blouse—worn alone or peeking out from under a crew neck sweater or cardigan, cutesy allover prints reminiscent of the 1950s, a time when life seemed simpler, silhouettes were pulled together, and television became a factor in dictating popular fashion styles.

Television icon Lucille Ball is another strong style setter for the indie girl because of her quirky but feminine clothing choices and boisterous personality. *I Love Lucy* hit American television screens in 1951 and still runs globally in syndication today. Ball's eye-catching, fiery red hair mirrored her wacky personality and crazy antics. Her clothing came second to her onscreen persona, but it echoed her upbeat spirit and also captured popular clothing styles of the 1950s.

The quirky-yet-pulled-together look is still seen among the indie set today, most often as oversized cat-eye eyeglasses or the crimson-hued hair color popular with girls who love the spunky red shade made iconic by the comedienne.

Ball's hair was dyed from her natural blond to a ginger shade in order to match her lively personality. Red is still popular with indie girls as well as Southern California's strong rockabilly community, which sports victory rolls and 50s-inspired ponytails as well as pinup girl–inspired dresses.

The rockabilly contingency in LA encompasses more than just a passion for the upbeat music; it's a subculture heavily steeped in an entire lifestyle that includes a thriving custom-car scene and a strong focus on fashion.

For rockabilly girls, this means short, blunt bangs, 40s and 50s silhouettes like knee-length pencil skirts, Capri-length pants, and body-hugging ensembles reminiscent of original pinup girls. Also, stacked heels and ultra-feminine frame bags become edgy and more modern when mixed with a smattering of colorful tattoos, also inspired by the 50s and car culture. For men, it's a mix of Southern California punk and classic 50s greaser, with slicked-back hair or a pompadour, cuffed dark jeans and a white T-shirt or retro bowling shirt.

While the rockabilly look turns up the volume on 50s style, Ball's cinched-waist, full-skirt dresses, embellished shirt collars, and prim pearl necklaces represented a more polished aspect of the era that also informs indie girls of today. The Beatniks from the beachside area of Venice are also an indie eclectic influencing–subculture, but a much more subdued scene, with less of a focus on fashion that in its own way contributed to the rich backdrop against which so much of today's LA indie style is drawn.

Though it may be known for a colorful, bustling boardwalk, modern million-dollar beach houses, and, more recently, food trucks and trendy farm-to-table-style eateries, 1950s Venice Beach was home to LA's beatnik contingency, who converged in the breezy seaside coffee shops and tiny bookstores that peppered the then-much-grittier locale.

New York had Greenwich Village and San Francisco had North Beach. Southern California's landing spot for the beat generation—nestled right against the ocean—was decidedly less metropolitan.

Fashion wasn't a priority to the beat generation, who donned simple black silhouettes, minimal jewelry, and beanies as a way of separating themselves from the mainstream, often coming off more like theater stagehands, who blend into the shadows of a performance.

For women, the beatnik look entailed flats (ballet-style flats and skimmer-type shoes), and an Audrey Hepburn–esque gamine look of pencil skirts and turtlenecks.

The look was the antithesis of what was happening in mainstream fashion at the time. Beatnik women didn't wear the coiffed hair, pinched waists, and full skirts of those who were donning Dior in the 1950s. They refused conventions, both politically and sartorially, sporting flatter, more natural hair and generally doing the opposite of what was happening with high-end French fashion that was popular during the decade.

But even if the look was understated, it still carried with it a strong sense of style that has influenced clothing in film (*Funny Face* and *The Subterraneans*) as well as the dance costumes worn by Martha Graham's dance company, which included round necklines and full skirts. Male dancers were dressed in plain black pants and black turtlenecks. Short cropped bangs, hair pulled up into a high ponytail, pedal pusher pants, a cigarette dangling from the lips, and solid simple dresses with circle skirts (sans petticoats) were style staples of the women who surrounded the beatnik scene in LA. Pioneering American sportswear designers Claire McCardell and Bonnie Cashin were also heavily influenced by the simple lines and more understated approach to dressing that was prominent among the subculture.

Coffee houses were an integral part of the beatnik scene, as people would gather for readings or to rap about ideas and poets. The Venice West Cafe was the main hangout and hub of the Venice beatnik scene. Opened in 1958 by poet Stuart Perkoff, who turned an old bleach factory on Dudley Avenue into what he envisioned as a bustling coffee house for the locals, the place is described by John Arthur Maynard in his book *Venice West: The Beat Generation in Southern California* as having patrons who were racially mixed and shabby-looking, furniture that was basic and primitive, and walls that were covered with slogans and abstract paintings.

A defunct bingo parlor housed another bustling locale for the beatnik contingency of LA. The Gas House, located in the heart of Venice on Ocean Front Walk, was a space for art exhibitions and poetry readings, and also hosted an open mike night, much to the chagrin of nonbeatnik Venice residents who tried to close down the club.

A couple of decades after the beatniks claimed Venice as their stomping ground, the area also became home to thrift stores frequented by people in similar fringe subcultures long before thrift shopping or vintage clothing was socially acceptable and certainly before it became fashionable.

LA's indie look is a nod to decades past, put together with a drop of irony and irreverence. Vintage pieces, worn more literally or mixed with an edgy aesthetic, all work to create a colorful and unique style, inspired by the independent spirits rooted in the cultural history of LA.

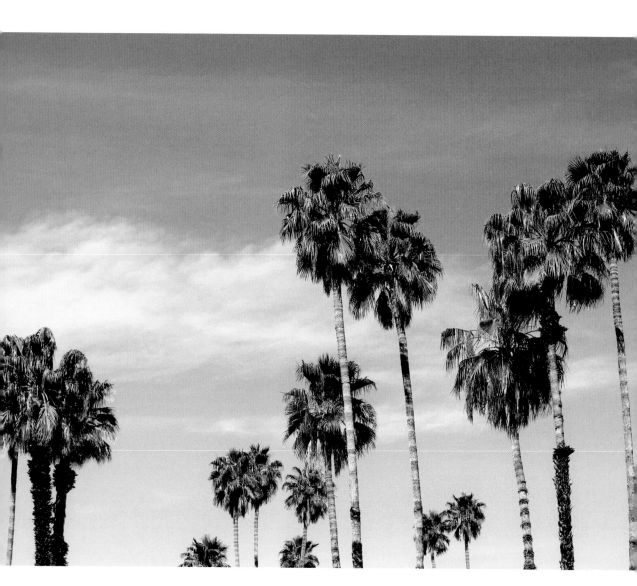

WHITNEY PORT

LA style is a reflection of your character. As a born-and-raised Angeleno, it is quite easy for me to feel confident and comfortable with a T-shirt and jeans, yet the look and feel of such pieces are what you are able to make your own. Whether you are a beach babe, an artist, a lady who lunches, or an actress, all we really want here in LA is to be comfortable. The sun's presence allows us to be free-flowing and casual—just the way I like it.

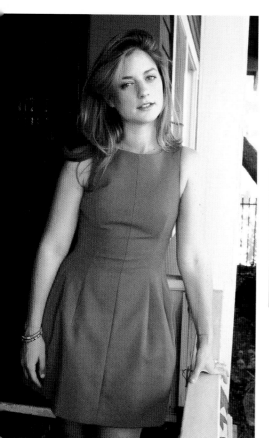

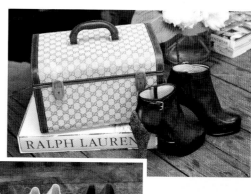

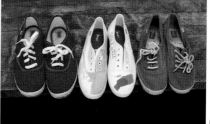

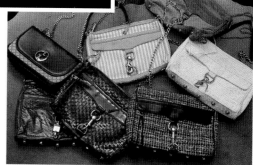

Name: ILARIA URBINATI   Hometown: Rome, Italy
Occupation: STYLIST and Retailer

How would you describe your style?

I definitely dress in theme and there's always a story to where my looks come from. I use clothes to create a make-believe. One minute I might want to pretend I'm living on a ranch, wearing a white button-up and equestrian boots and the next minute I want to be Winona Ryder in *Reality Bites*, wearing a grungy red T-shirt or floral baby-doll dresses.

What inspires how you dress?

Movies (and sometimes television) are always an inspiration. It can be any movie or something totally silly like old episodes of 90210 to simple 70s war-era looks like Jane Fonda in *Coming Home*.

Do you have any clothing or accessory items you wear daily or almost daily?

I pretty much live in Keds. That's one of the virtues of LA weather. Plus, they make me feel like Liv Tyler in *Stealing Beauty* or Jennifer Grey in *Dirty Dancing*.

Who are your favorite designers?

Ralph Lauren, Calvin Klein, Proenza Schouler, Christopher Kane, Burberry, Dolce & Gabbana, Erdem, Isabel Marant.

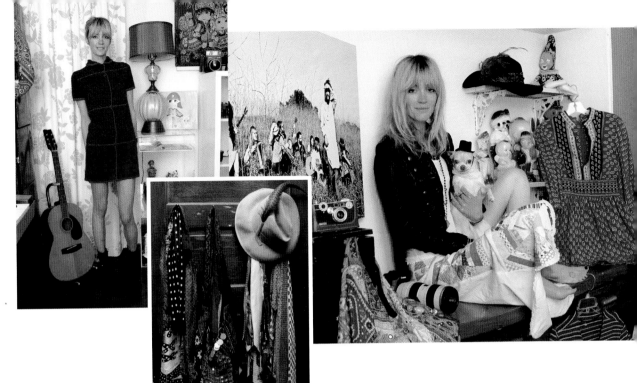

Name: **JULIE LING**   Hometown: LOS ANGELES, CA
Occupation: Renaissance Artisan

How would you describe your style?
If I could compare my style to a mood ring, I'd say the colors span from hippie to mod to Victorian circus.

Who are your style icons?
My grandmother Beatrice Ling was the most elegant woman I have ever met. She is my muse. Her beauty and grace inspired my first photograph. Her style reflected her heart.

What are your go-to pieces in your closet?
I love my grandfather's Pennington tan hat, my mom's long maxiskirt from the 60s with patchwork embroidery, and the miniskirt I made from a hand-stitched authentic Baltic long skirt of sashes that I bought off a divorced hippie couple from Latvia, my black Costume National ankle boots from 1999, and my ringmaster-shaped leather jacket.

What would you consider a signature aspect of your style?
A 60s-style mod dress would be my signature piece of clothing.

What is the last thing you bought?
The last thing I bought was a vintage skirt from the 50s with pencil-drawn clowns on the bottom half.

Who are your favorite designers?
I have a hard time following anything specific. I like things that are recycled mostly.

Name your signature scent, hairstyle, hair color, or other things you feel distinguish your style.
People always say I smell like donuts or chocolate chip cookies. One of my eyes is green and I always have bangs.

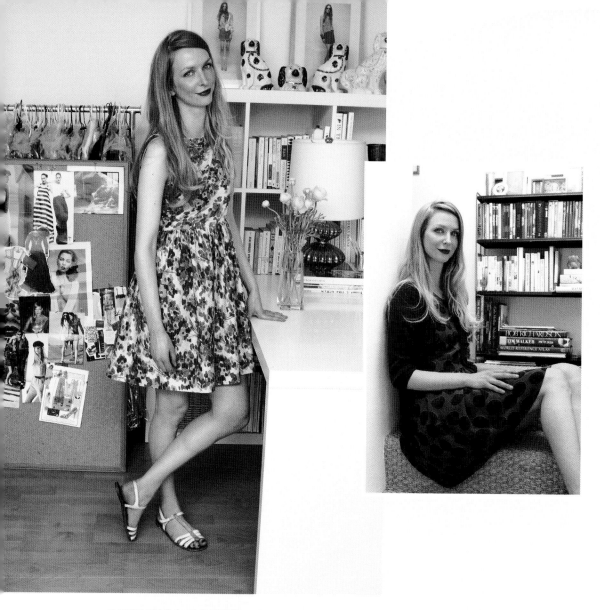

Name: MELISSA COKER   Hometown: Lake Forest, IL   Occupation: Designer

How would you describe your style?
Rosemary Woodhouse meets Margot Tenenbaum. My style is girlish prep.

What or who inspires you to get dressed and shop?
Friends, girls on the street, movies like *Shampoo*, magazines like *Lula*.

What are your go-to pieces and/or your favorite item in your closet? And what would you consider a signature aspect of your style?

Chanel two-tone flats, Chanel 2.55 purse, and Hermès Medor watch. They make everything look nicer.

Who are your favorite designers?
Wren, Charles Anastase, Chanel, Jason Wu.

Name your signature scent, hairstyle, hair color, or other things you feel distinguish your style.
Perfume: Costes. Hairstyle: bed head.

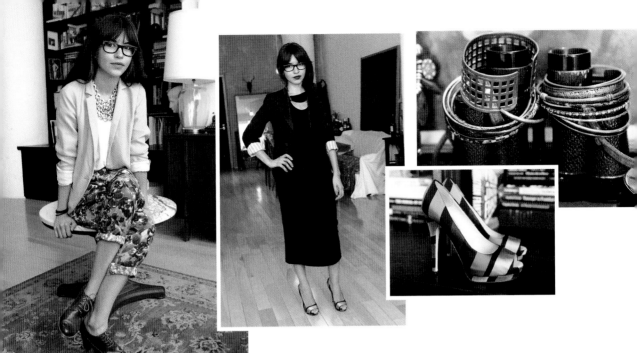

Name: **ERIN BARAJAS** **Hometown:** MONTEBELLO, CA

Occupation: TRADE SHOW PRODUCER

How would you describe your style?

My style is probably most accurately described as "middle-child modern," because I wear pared-down secondhand and vintage staples every day. As the middle child, I grew up wearing a lot of hand-me-downs and I guess I never stopped. I love clothes with a history or a story.

What is your favorite item in your closet? And what would you consider a signature aspect of your style?

My favorite item in my closet is a full black leather skirt I snagged while in Paris on my honeymoon. I wear it when I'm feeling superfancy. Blazers, jackets, and coats are my go-to workhorses. I wear them constantly, with everything. Current favorites are a dove-gray men's blazer cut from glove leather by Corpus (so many hidden pockets!), a vintage boy's Oscar de la Renta tux jacket with tails, and a shrunken Bebe jacket that I bought ten years ago.

Describe your signature hairstyle.

My hair, which on good days is a little beachy and on bad days looks like a Fraggle [Rock character], is prematurely graying—which I love. I'm anxiously awaiting a full-fledged Mrs. Robinson streak, but until then I stick to two "styles": down in a chaotic riot of frizz or up in a huge top-knot. Big hair, it's not just for New Jersey.

Do you have any items you wear daily or almost daily?

My eyesight is pitiful, so I wear glasses every day and they've become my signature. For the last two years I've been superloyal to a chunky pair of nerd frames. When I bought them I demanded a pair of Clark Kent–style glasses and I guess I got what I asked for. The only other thing I wear with the same regularity is my engagement ring. My husband had a blue-green sapphire solitaire made for me and I love its watery color.

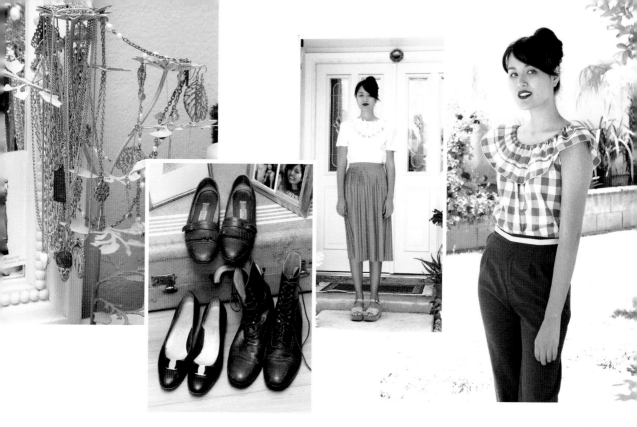

Name: **ASHLEY BALAYUT**   **Hometown:** Irvine, CA
Occupation: Vintage Clothing Seller and Photo Archivist

How would you describe your style?
Playful, comfortable, and unpredictable.

What inspires your style?
In a broad sense it would be history. I love gleaning inspiration from studying past times and seeing how people lived way back when. Also, growing up in Southern California, the influence of the skate/surf culture is undeniable.

What would you consider a signature aspect of your style?
While I do dress fairly boyish, I'm also known for dressing quite feminine. I collect vintage dresses in a variety of colors, cuts, and prints. No era is off limits.

What is the last thing you bought? And what is your must-have piece of clothing right now?
A pair of brown leather flat lace-up boots and a pair of 1970s brown penny loafers

both purchased at the Goodwill. As far as a must-have piece of clothing, colorful socks (thin stripes are a favorite) can add a bit of intrigue to the plainest outfit.

Who are your favorite designers?
I'm not really into designer clothing (I buy 80 percent of what I wear from thrift stores and flea markets), but aesthetically I do appreciate Marc Jacobs and Erin Fetherston.

What is your signature hairstyle? And what other things do you feel distinguish your style?
Oversized vintage grandpa cardigans. I'd wear one with every outfit if I could. Besides that, I feel like my hair is sort of a signature. It's never been dyed and it's just so long, when I wear it down I feel like I'm wearing a statement accessory.

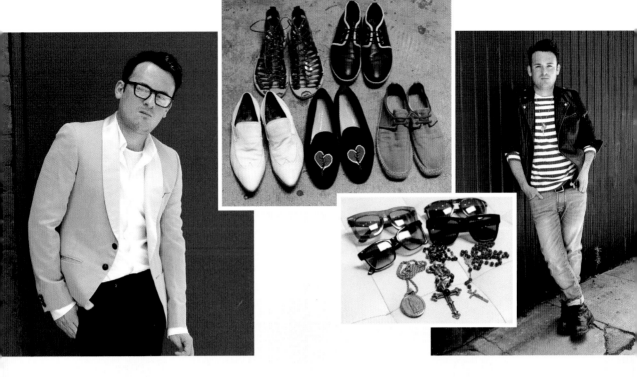

Name: **MIKE VARGAS**   Hometown: LOS ANGELES, CA
Occupation: FASHION PUBLICIST

How would you describe your style?

It changes every day and has never been constant. I might feel like being preppy one day and the next I'm in jeans and a torn shirt and in slacks and a blazer the next. Not sure if it's a way of being defiant of fashion trends but I like it!

Do you have any style icons?

I grew up in Hollywood so there's no way of getting around the influence of old Hollywood actors. There's something extremely timeless and sexy about the way Brando, Dean, McQueen dressed that's still very relevant. But I also love the modern-day dandy, like Patrick McDonald and the late Sebastian Horsley. And then there's the always-dashing Tom Ford, whose film *A Single Man* inspired me on various levels after watching it.

What are the go-to pieces in your closet? What would you consider a signature aspect of your style?

My go-to pieces at the moment are a black distressed denim jacket by Surface to Air and a gold charm necklace with various religious medals and a huge 1940s Italian crucifix. I wear the necklace almost every day. As far as signature aspects of my style, I would say that layering is a big part of it. I love to layer.

What is the last thing you bought?

Last thing I bought was a pair of chukka boots from Vintage Shoe Company and a pair of espadrilles, both of which I will be wearing all summer. I'm a bit of a shoe fanatic.

Who are your favorite designers and your go-to places to shop?

My taste in designers is across the board. I love Shipley & Halmos, Dior Homme, Boris Bidjan Saberi, RAD by Rad Hourani, Ksubi Jeans, Dunhill, Trovata, Shades of Grey, Tom Ford, and a bit of vintage. In LA, I really like shopping at Confederacy. It's a great men's store.

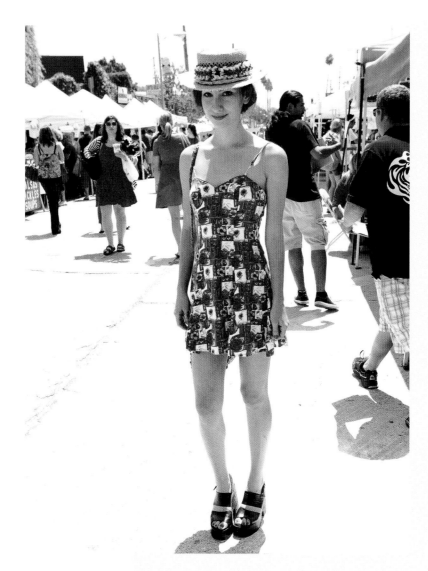

Name: DEANNE DESTLER   Hometown: LOS ANGELES, CA   Occupation: ACTRESS

How would you describe your style?
Decade tourist. Wandering farm girl in the city.

Do you have any style icons or count any films as inspiration?
Lillian Gish, my friends, *Lolita*.

What is the last thing you bought?
A large case of green tea.

Do you have a signature scent?
Dried gardenias, sunshine, post–dance floor aroma, Tom's of Maine (the less I shower the more I get complimented on how good I smell).

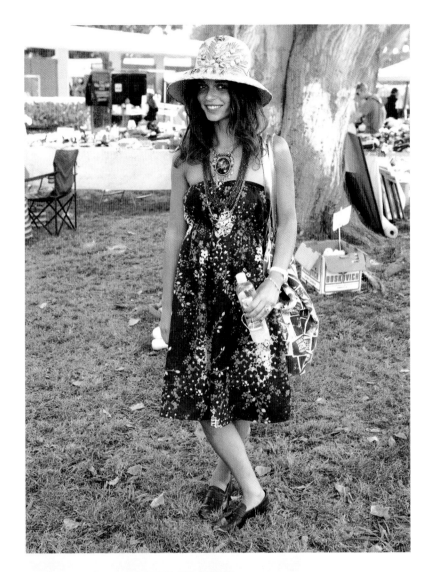

Name: **JUSTINE DEMEAUX**   Hometown: Paris, France
Occupation: FILM Production Intern

How would you describe your style?
  Hippie chic.

Do you have any style icons?
  Brigitte Bardot, Alice Dellal, Audrey
  Tautou, Georgia May Jagger.

What would you consider a signature aspect of your style?
  My necklaces.

What is the last thing you bought?
  Vintage sunglasses.

Who are your favorite designers?
  Pierre Cardin.

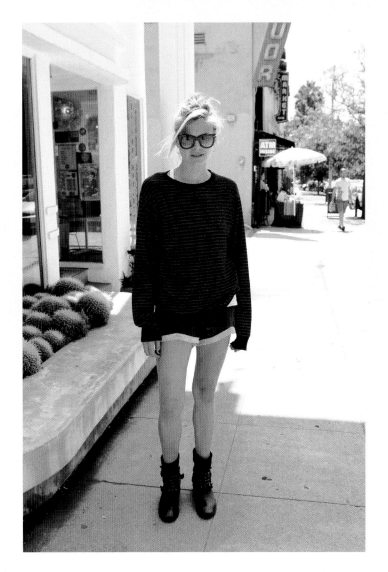

Name: ELIZA COUPE   Hometown: LOS Angeles, CA   Occupation: Actress

How would you describe your style?
Edgy hipster-y.

Do you have any style icons?
The French do it all right. But right now I'm really into Diane Kruger's style and Alexa Chung's style. Chloe Sevigny and Kate Moss have also always been ones to watch for tips too. And of course those damn Olsen twins have always known what's up.

What are your go-to pieces and/or your favorite item in your closet?
My boots. All of my boots.

What is the last thing you bought?
I just bought a pair of Thierry Lasry sunglasses . . . and ordered another pair from his fall collection. Best sunglasses ever made.

Who are your favorite designers?
Big fan of vintage Chanel, Prada, the classics. I also love Sonia Rykiel, Isabel Marant, some Valentino, Alexander Wang . . . I could go on, but we'd be here awhile.

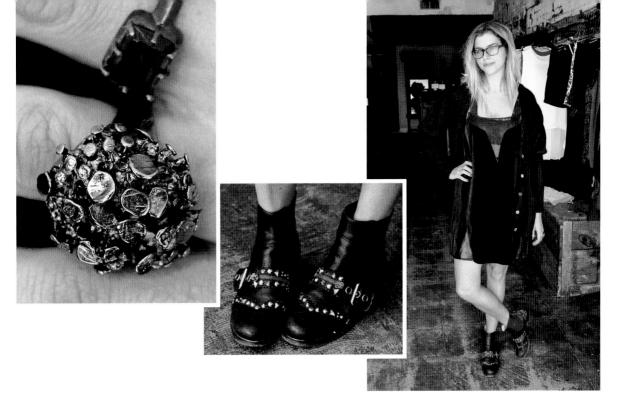

Name: MICHELLE VON BAUER   **Hometown:** ORANGE COUNTY, CA
Occupation: FREELANCE FASHION STYLIST

How would you describe your style?
Eclectic, effortless, edgy. I like to mix high and low pieces, vintage and new, soft and hard. I put things together depending on my mood of the moment—so it could be jeans and a basic T, or mixed prints and textures.

Do you have any style icons or count any films as inspiration?
I admire girls on the street with their own sense of fashion who aren't afraid to mix and match and take risks. Women like Alexa Chung, Erin Wasson, and Kate Moss.

What are your go-to pieces and your favorite item in your closet? And what would you consider a signature aspect of your style?
I have currently been wearing my Miu Miu boots and Rick Owens leather jacket with everything during the week. And my glasses are a signature! Also, chunky cardigans, ripped jean shorts, and blouses are standard pieces in my closet. And *a lot* of black!

What is the last thing you bought?
A vintage dress from the flea market! I love thrifting.

Who are your favorite designers?
Theysken's Theory, Alexander Wang, Proenza Schouler, Phillip Lim, Isabel Marant, and Givenchy.

What are your beauty habits?
I am pretty low-maintenance during the day. I rarely dye or style my hair, but if I want to get a little more dressed up at night, I'm all about the loose, messy wave. My skin is very sensitive, so I have to wear a really good face and eye cream. Nude Skincare is simply amazing. It's organic with probiotics that works with your body's natural chemistry. I love the fresh face look with either a black cat eye or a statement lip.

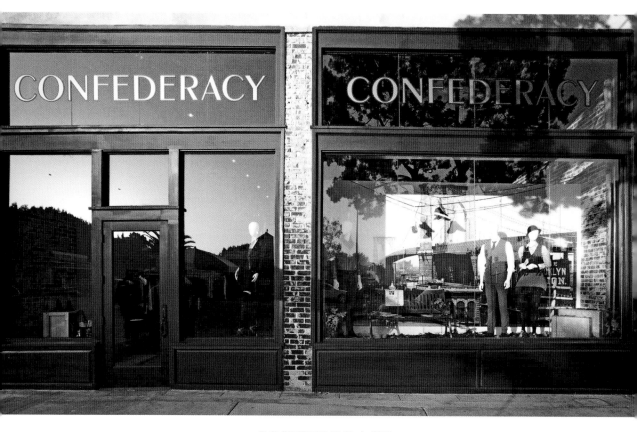

CONFEDERACY
4661 Hollywood Blvd.
Los Angeles, CA 90027
(323) 913-3040

Across town from the jumbo mall and ritzy boutiques of Beverly Hills sits a space that apart from high-end and contemporary labels such as Proenza Schouler, Alexander Wang, and 3.1 Phillip Lim, might have you fooled it was a quaint bookstore straight out of the 1940s.

Stylist and store co-owner Ilaria Urbinati dresses celebrities and edits her shop with the same keen eye and attention to detail as when she is pulling pieces for her famous clients. She also considers the specific way women in Los Angeles dress and

shop. "The number one thing for girls in LA is comfort," she says.

Urbinati buys pieces from Proenza Schouler and Thakoon that can be thrown on with ease and worn with denim, so they become wardrobe staples that women can essentially live in. "I'll pair a tweed jacket with ripped jeans, so there's that nice play of opposites," she says. "If LA girls wear something dressy they pair it with something casual. There's this high and low effect that's everywhere, but more so here."

Sticking to her stylist sensibilities, Ur-

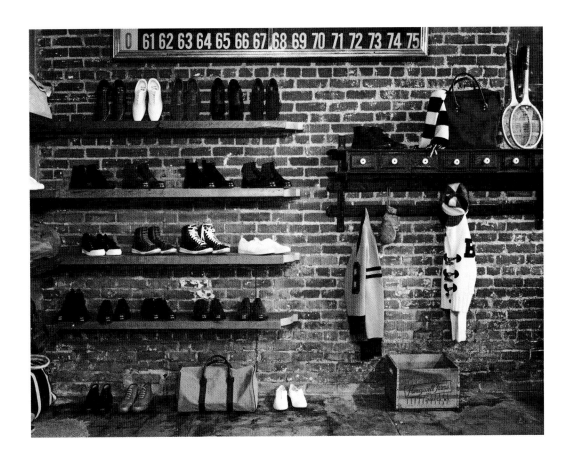

binati curates the store with pieces that can't be found everywhere and buys according to style moments in time such as 1970s Brooke Shields, 1990s grunge and even old photos of her mother, who she brands as having "really sick style." "I'm a very referential person," says Urbinati. "I buy in a certain way that the customer definitely feels like they are being styled by me."

And that includes the guys too. Connected by an airy outdoor patio is a space in the back of the brick-and-concrete store that houses menswear as well as the shoe section, featuring sky-high heels from Guiseppe Zanotti and an extensive collection of lace-up oxfords and canvas sneakers from F-Troupe and Keds.

"Girls here want to be comfortable," says Urbinati. "They definitely cycle in trends but within a comfort zone." This is why in addition to oxford flats she hangs drapey, fleece and jersey pieces from Monrow and stretchy denim leggings from Goldsign and Acne among the designer items. But don't expect the floaty floor-length bohemian pieces people generally associate with LA. "Even though LA has that bohemian thing, I hate the word and I don't buy bohemian," she says. "But there still is that feeling and I try and translate bohemian in other ways."

That said, Urbinati's golden rule is to stock her store with the most covetable and to-die-for pieces that inspire people to be creative storytellers with the way they dress. "At the end of the day I buy something that's really stunning. There's no set rule. You just have to be freaking out over it."

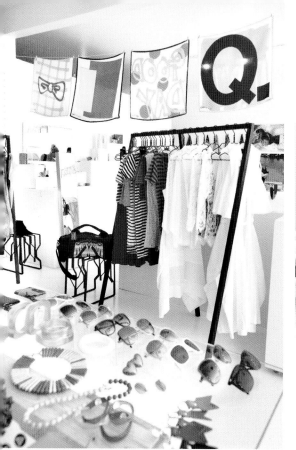

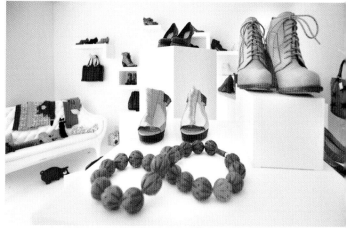

TENOVERSIX

8425 Melrose Ave.
Los Angeles, CA 90069
(323) 330-9355

New York transplant designer Kristen Lee has an eye for the unexpected. Just the thing her friends and customers—an impressive mix of stylists, fashion editors, and taste makers—look for when trying to find a to-die-for pair of shoes that are more likely to be from brands like Surface to Air or Rachel Comey than Christian Louboutin or Jimmy Choo. "We wanted to cater more to the 'transplant' contingent of LA," says Lee. "The people we know who have moved to LA from Manhattan, Brooklyn, San Francisco, London, or Paris and who already know most of our designers and 'get' our concept and mix of merchandise."

Appropriately named after the numbers scrawled on a scrap of paper sticking out of the Mad Hatter's top hat in *Alice's Adventures in Wonderland*, the store is a whimsical mix of shoes, jewelry, limited edition clothing and bags, and coffee table and art books that evoke a feeling of sartorial wonder and discovery. Lee was inspired to open TenOverSix upon relocating to Los Angeles from New York. Instantly falling in love with the relaxed and escapist nature of the city, she wanted to contribute to that notion.

Along with her business partner, Brady Cunningham, Lee has curated an

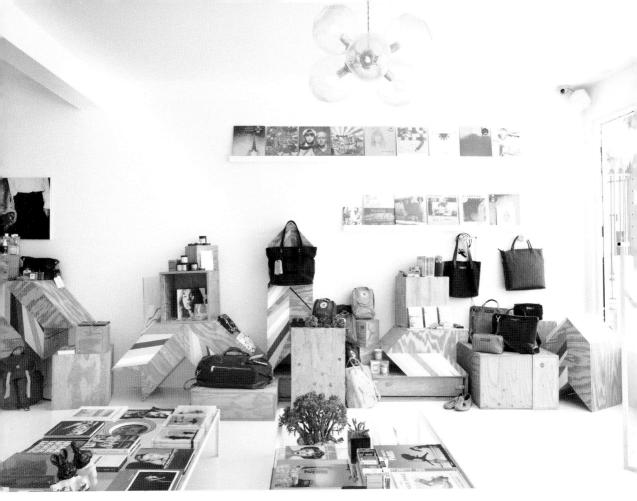

accessory-heavy boutique that is nestled next to Diane von Furstenberg and Marc Jacobs in West Hollywood. The store was born in the fall of 2008 out of what Lee and Cunningham saw as a gap in the LA retail market for up-and-coming, harder-to-find, and limited edition items that Angelenos certainly have a palate for but count on picking up on travels to Paris, London, or Tokyo. "We wanted to bring a bit of that more fashion-y, independent, small label, and artistic sensibility to the Los Angeles retail scene," says Lee.

Now these wares, which in the past were mainly carried at Japanese and European boutiques, are accessible to LA girls who appreciate labels beyond the ones they can find at every department store. They look to TenOverSix as a go-to spot for edgy and interesting accessories to mix into their casual chic uniform of tap shorts, vintage dresses, tailored black or navy blue blazers, and nautical-inspired striped shirts.

What Lee refers to as "smart, detailed, and a bit tongue-in-cheek designers" such as Slow and Steady Wins the Race, Vena Cava, Bodkin, and LD Tuttle are housed in the store as well as Lee and Cunningham's TenOverSix private label, which the designers describe as "chic day dresses, simple bags, and the everyday pieces we want to wear most."

Judging by the cool-girl contingents that frequent their shop, they're not alone.

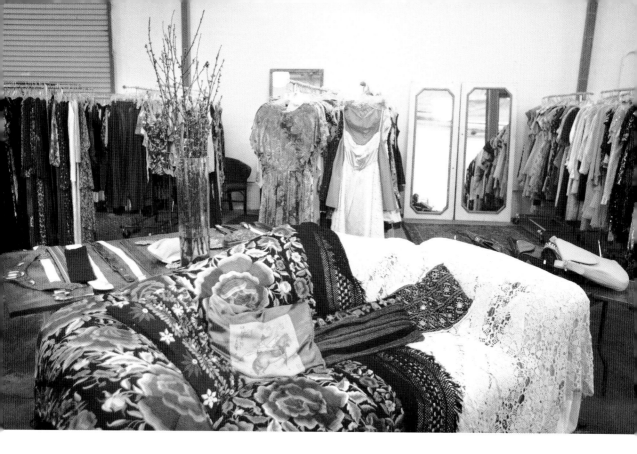

SHAREEN VINTAGE

1721 N. Spring St.
Los Angeles, CA 90012
(323) 276-6226

Judging by Shareen Mitchell's vault of vintage wares, which are always in demand by LA girls in the know, you would assume the former *Vogue* magazine staffer has been hoarding and archiving hard-to-find gems for the past several decades. But the owner of Shareen Vintage has had quite a colorful road to retail, and her background as a model scout, fashion editor, stylist, and actress have equipped her with an arsenal of skills (which include an impeccable eye for what trendy girls want to wear) for opening one of the best-kept shopping secrets in Los Angeles.

Mitchell began her road to retail in 2003 after noticing that the runways

were teeming with strong vintage references. "That was the year that Marc Jacobs for Louis Vuitton, Chloé, and Dior sent dresses down the runway that had a true waist," says Mitchell. "Everyone was doing past decades. And at that point everyone was wearing vintage for vintage sake, but not using it to be as fashionable as what was on the runway at the moment."

She initially spent eighty dollars on thrift store dresses from the 1970s and 1950s that were comparable to the looks walking down the runways that season and rented a booth at the Melrose Trading Post flea market. As one of two vintage clothing stalls at the market, Mitchell quickly

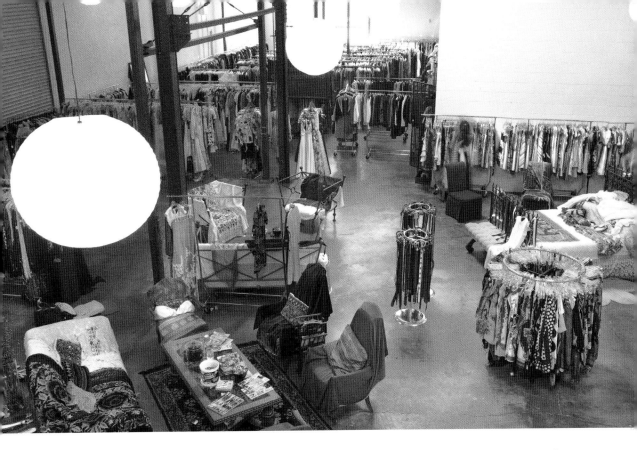

became the go-to person for affordable and on-trend vintage dresses that she was selling to fashion-savvy girls for just twenty-four dollars. "The fashion girls were the ones who appreciated it," says Mitchell. "They abandoned their baggy jeans and started wearing dresses."

Mitchell's styling and magazine background also set her apart from what anyone was doing as she would rework pieces and style them with leather belts, corsets, and ribbons, showing women how to update vintage and make it their own.

Shareen Vintage soon left the Melrose Trading Post and moved to an out-of-the-way downtown LA warehouse that was initially open only a couple of days a week and took an accurate GPS system and a hunger for affordable vintage to find. The first day Mitchell's brick-and-mortar store was open for business, a line full of

her flea market followers formed down the block. Soon the celebrities who also knew her from the market started coming to check out her expanded stash of clothing. Katie Holmes, Victoria Beckham, Kirsten Dunst, and Katy Perry would come to pick up armloads of her well-edited selection.

Mitchell has a strict no-boys-allowed policy in her store, which lets women comfortably try clothing on in the large open space and fosters the feeling of a sample sale-meets-vintage-lovers club. Every day, women head to the outskirts of downtown to check out the racks of mostly skirts, dresses, and camisoles stocked inside the store. "The location is part of the cachet," says Mitchell. "My regular customers say, 'Shareen's is like *Fight Club*. You don't talk about *Fight Club*.' "

Word has certainly gotten out due to the trendsetters who have been shopping her store for the past couple years, and Mitchell has since been tapped to do projects and collaborations with stores like Madewell. She also gathers pieces for specific high-end designers to reference when they come to town. "I source for designers and pull for them," she says. "As I'm buying I put things aside for design-ers and show it to them when they come in. It's nice to be part of something bigger, something more mainstream."

With a strong following of trendsetters and celebrities, the once-word-of-mouth shopping destination is no longer so hush-hush, but it also shows no signs of losing its cachet.

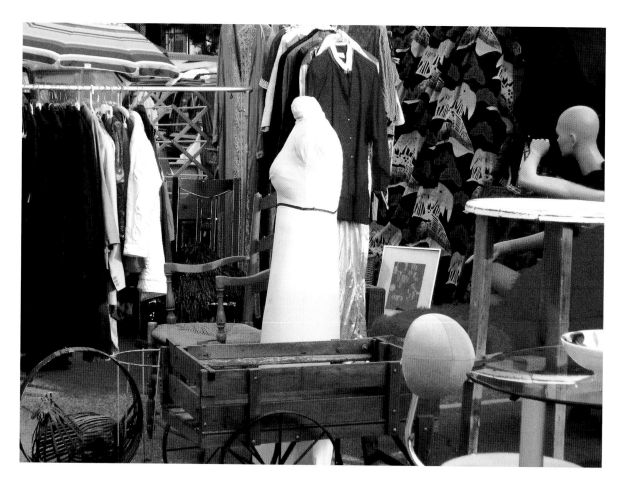

MELROSE TRADING POST
7850 Melrose Ave.
Los Angeles, CA 90046
(323) 655-7679

Most major flea markets have shed their reputation for housing chintzy knickknacks and random throwaways. Rather, they've become cool and often hipster heavy, catering to those who seek out salvaged and reworked secondhand furniture, 70s knee-high boots, and local jewelry from designers who are just starting out. The Melrose Trading Post is LA's most accessible and least overwhelming flea market, where you can stroll through in a couple of hours browsing vintage clothing, handmade soaps, old records, and reupholstered chairs.

The market is set up every Sunday in the parking lot of Fairfax High School, which sits on a busy corner of Melrose and Fairfax Avenue. Besides selling trendy and interesting finds to shoppers each weekend, the event raises money for the high school's various academic and extracurricular programs.

A two-dollar entrance fee grants you access to peruse and haggle amid the merchandise or relax and grab something to eat in the flea market's no-frills food market.

But it's generally the accessories that shine the brightest at the Melrose Trading Post. Vendors selling both new and old pieces have strong displays of their work or a nicely curated selection of jewelry from the 1970s and 80s. Nothing too precious, but definitely fun and easy to buy and work into a wardrobe for styling purposes.

Groups of girls come to the market post-brunch or some stroll in solo clutching a large cup of coffee. They're always dressed to be seen, but in the most disheveled and devil-may-care kind of way. They wear vintage dresses with lace-up leather boots and sometimes sport a quirky sun hat that looks like it belonged to a crazy aunt, so whether you're shopping or just strolling, the people-watching can be as intriguing as the merchandise.

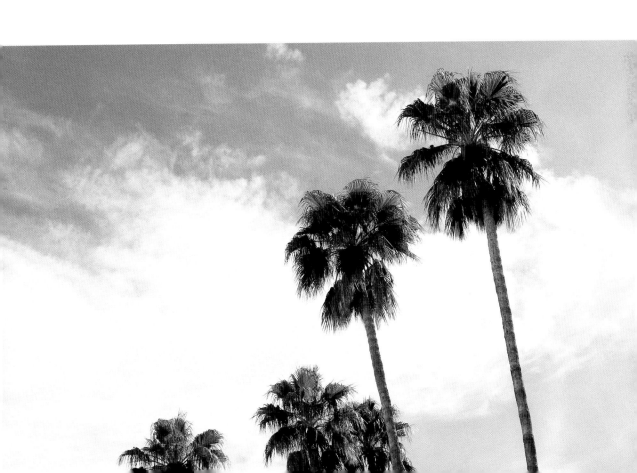

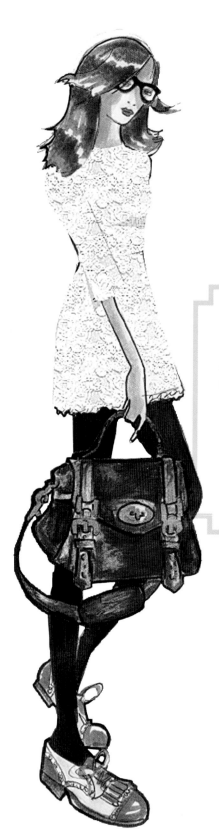

HOW TO GET THE LOOK
indie eclectic

Indie girls wear vintage silhouettes with
modern-day flair, pairing kicky dresses
with tomboy staples like lace-up oxfords
and chunky eyewear.

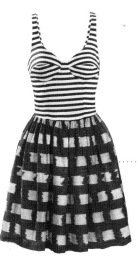
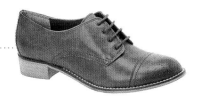
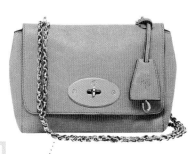
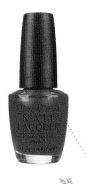
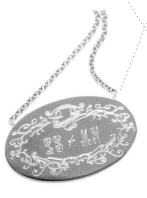
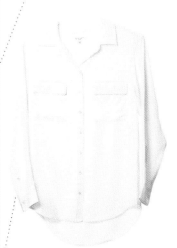
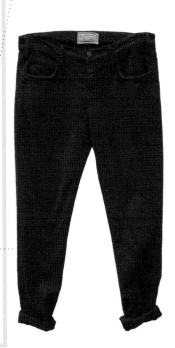

A retro-inspired dress done in a cute and girlie print is a definite indie staple.

The indie twist is in the mix of accessories, like menswear-inspired leather oxfords and delicate, feminine jewelry.

A vintage-inspired satchel is bookish but stylish.

Sweet-looking and sentimental-feeling jewelry worn alone or layered softens up the tomboy vibe.

A fitted heather-gray blazer pairs well over a dress or with rolled-up jeans.

Chunky eyeglasses are an indie girl and guy go-to accessory.

Nail polish doesn't always have to be a traditionally girly shade. An offbeat hue adds a modern twist to vintage clothing.

A boyfriend-style button-down blouse looks adorable tucked into a pleated skirt or worn under a tailored blazer.

Colored denim gives any outfit an interesting and unexpected pop.

Berry-stained lips add to a doll-like appeal.

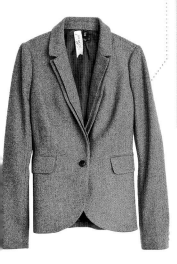
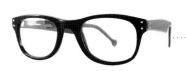
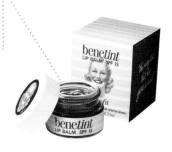

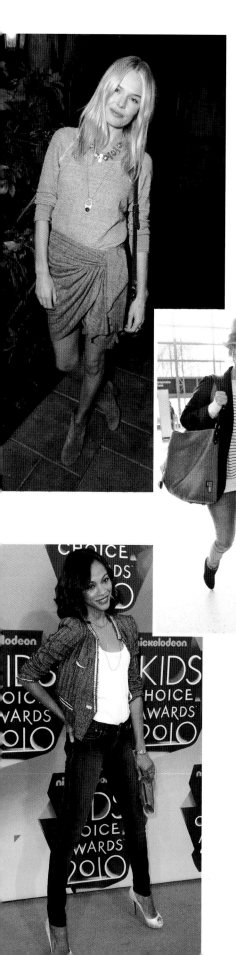

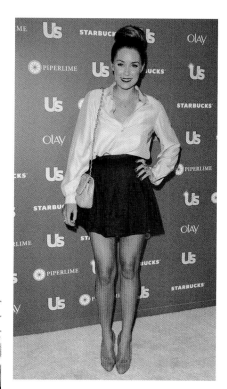

Clockwise from top left: **Kate Bosworth** attends an awards season party at Chateau Marmont in 2011. **Lauren Conrad** at *Us Weekly*'s 2011 Hot Hollywood Party in Hollywood. **Nicole Richie** attends a Coachella BBQ thrown by Mulberry at the Parker Palm Springs. Actress **Zoe Saldana** arrives at Nickelodeon's 23rd Annual Kid's Choice Awards at UCLA's Pauley Pavilion, March 27, 2010, Los Angeles. **Rachel Bilson** departs from LAX in 2010.

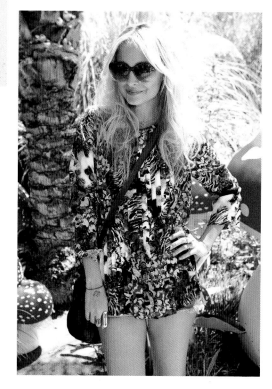

casual chic

LA girls have an ease to their style. They love cool fabric in all types of jersey that mix well with the tough side of denim or washed leather. They adopt a carefree attitude by day but can easily transform by night for a cocktail or a walk down the red carpet.

—CATHERINE MALANDRINO

The modern LA girl or guy is a master of taking celebrity-style, high fashion, and mass-market trends, mixing them together, and wearing the look in a way that is unique to the eclectic atmosphere, abundant sunshine, and laid-back attitude of the city. The resulting look is casual chic: an effortless blend of fashion-driven style that's never fussy or overdone.

The current-day look of LA doesn't point to the past as much as it takes contemporary trends from the runway and the street and puts them together—all with signature West Coast ease.

Take for example the innerwear as outerwear trend of spring 2009 that was seen in the collections of Dior, Balenciaga, and Marc Jacobs. Dior did a polished interpretation, sending out 40s film noir–style via sheer bow-neck blouses tucked into body-hugging pencil skirts, delicate black bras peeking through—adding a harder, sexier edge to the soft silhouette. Marc Jacobs showed delicate satin bras—worn on the outside of shirts—as well as layered underpinnings that drew a quiet contrast to all the ruffled trims festooning his collection that season.

Months later, the trend popped up all over LA— but it had been filtered through a Southern California–style siphon, morphing into something fresh and different. Ultimately, it was a prime example of how trend-conscious girls in LA translate designer fashion through their own cultural viewpoint.

SoCal girls sported oversize T-shirts with gaping arm holes that dipped down to the bottom of their rib cages, layered over hot pink, purple, or black bras that peeked out in the same way the 40s-style underpinnings did on the Dior runway, but with a twist that was both sporty, relaxed, and much more liberated.

This combo was often paired with jeans or jean shorts, flip-flops or classic ballet flats—tempering the edgier styling of visible lace underwear that was happening up top.

It was a prime example of how LA's style-savvy set from West Side high school kids to off duty celebrities reinterpret current-day ideas in fashion and apply them to the city's eclectic atmosphere. The twist on trendy looks is always casual, free, and steeped in personal self-expression—and paired with a flair and exuberance for accessorizing.

Take, for instance, beaded leather bracelets comingling with Cartier watches and ratty pieces of string on the tanned arms of celebrities and civilians alike. High-fashion trends are tempered with tees, denim, sandals, and slightly disheveled accessories, spinning the big ideas into something more befitting of the light, landscape, and lifestyle that is LA. A blazer or leather jacket thrown over a frilly dress is the norm in a city where formality is, for the most part, a foreign concept.

And while there are countless stylish LA women who embody a Southern California casual-chic look, certain celebrities stand out for consistently mixing high fashion with West Coast casual, creating an inspiring template for girls all over the globe.

They are designer muses and off duty fashion poster girls who sit front row at a Chanel runway show and are on top of the latest collections from cult-fav labels like Isabel Marant, Celine, and Proenza Schouler. But they always manage to temper high-end inspira-

PHILLIP LIM

LA will always be my spiritual home, and I look back at my years spent there very fondly. I think I would be lying if I said my designs weren't influenced by the LA attitude towards life, the free-spirited, easy way that only really exists there. There is something about the LA state of mind that will always exist in my designs.

tion with toned-down pieces for a look that's easy, effortless, and a prime example of how designer pieces are styled for the West Coast lifestyle.

Rachel Bilson has become a style icon to millions of women all over the world and is now a brand ambassador for Sunglass Hut and gives style advice on online retailer Piperlime.com as well as in her monthly fashion column for *InStyle* magazine. Bilson has become known for her flair for pairing covetable high-end items with beat-up jeans and signature classic Ray-Ban Wayfarers. Her aesthetic is decidedly feminine and always very put together. Even her off duty look is adorable, whether she's walking her dog or running errands. And on the red carpet, she still maintains a beachy ease, wearing gowns, cocktail dresses, and jewelry that suit her tiny frame rather than overwhelming her.

Kate Bosworth's blend of basics and Parisian-inspired pieces leave the actress looking consistently elegant and perfectly playful at the same time. She wears music-festival chic as effortlessly as she does edgy ensembles when attending fashion shows, where she's become a front-row staple. (Bosworth's thin frame and fresh-scrubbed look make her a designer's dream to dress.) She's game to try new trends but always manages to style herself in a way that is classic and understated.

Lauren Conrad's style has become synonymous with the beachy Orange County lifestyle as much as it has the glamour of the red carpet. Conrad manages to look like a starlet, while still maintaining an approachable girl-next-door aesthetic that appeals to the fashion crowd as well as to college students, who identify with her innate ability to amp up typical California casual pieces into something more special, polished, and always superfeminine.

Nicole Richie, the ultimate boho babe, is well-known for being able to blend hippie chic with rock and designer trends, all without looking like a fashion victim. Whether she's in a tissue-thin T-shirt and bell bottoms or a long and colorful flowy dress and heels, her free-spirited nature and preference for including casual pieces, comes across in the way she layers accessories, her unique often 70s Elton John–esque sunglasses, and long beach-waved hair parted down the center.

Whether a look is heavy on the accessories, leans toward boho, or takes a subtle LA twist on a trend, the city by and large boasts a jeans and T-shirt uniform that on paper sounds ho-hum, but LA's top denim brands (among them, J Brand, 7 for All Mankind, and Paige Premium Denim) manage to elevate the classic jean to a level of premium quality and design that has redefined the idea of basics.

The city's influential denim scene has trickled up to the runways. Karl Lagerfeld even included jeans in his 2011 couture collection, breaking taboos in what constitutes couture. Celebrities including Cameron Diaz and Heidi Klum often team jeans with a Chanel jacket or silk blouse to red carpet movie premiers, proving that denim does belong on the red carpet when done right.

Recently, LA-based denim labels have collaborated with high-end designers on ultracoveted denim lines. J Brand collaborated with Hussein Chalayan and Christopher Kane on sleek and colorful denim, while Current/Elliott has turned out some edgy, fashion-forward designs with Marni.

That mix of high/low and juxtaposing very polished pieces with clean, more toned-down denim is a look that LA style setters thoroughly understand. Jeans are the perfect representation of the LA lifestyle—versatile, comfortable, and able to go from the beach to the office then dinner, all with the change of a shoe.

The city is home to the most innovative denim manufacturers in the world, and they approach dyeing and washing denim like brilliant mad scientists, constantly looking for the next best thing to improve fit, stretch, and wearability.

Adriano Goldschmied is the godfather of denim—not just in LA but globally. He created Diesel with Renzo Rosso as well as the Replay and Adriano Goldschmied brands and currently designs the Goldsign line, his latest denim endeavor. For the past thirteen years, Goldschmied has made LA his home and creative stomping grounds and spends four to five hours every day at his denim laundry in the outskirts of LA—overseeing the washing process and sanding treatments (all of which are done by hand). He calls LA the global epicenter of denim not only due to the know-how of its designers and manufacturers, but because the fabric itself has a long history in California.

Premium denim began to flourish in LA about a decade ago when many of the mass denim brands left the city for cheaper production in Mexico and China. People looking to manufacture more specialty premium denim had a prime opportunity to take over the resources the less expensive mass brands had left behind. A big hole remained, and premium denim designers stepped in and took over the abundant resources in order to create a new—and elevated—level of jeans that would eventually change how the world wears denim.

The thriving denim industry of LA isn't just about the manufacturing facilities. The city is home to a large and experienced body of talent that combines encyclopedic knowledge of denim with inspiration from the vibrant streets of Southern California.

Goldschmied counts people watching in Hollywood as a main inspiration for designing his denim line and for the creativity and wide swath of styles he observes when it comes to thinking of new design concepts.

The designers, manufacturing resources, lifestyle, weather, and glamour of Hollywood and access to celebrities are all elements Goldschmied feels make Los Angeles the prime place for creating (and wearing) a versatile staple like jeans. He also adds that the vintage pieces available in Los Angeles provide endless inspiration for denim designers looking to the past for "new" ideas.

"We can drive twenty minutes and be at the biggest flea market in the world [Rose Bowl Flea Market], when the competition is traveling fifteen hours to get there. All these things make what is happening here something that is really unique—a mix of things impossible to reproduce."

Jerome Dahan, creator and designer of Citizens of Humanity denim, echoes Goldschmied's sentiment saying that indeed LA is the capital of denim. Dahan's company has been among the top denim brands for the past decade, but his history in the industry proves equally as impressive. As a head designer of Guess and founder of 7 for all Mankind, Dahan has spent the past three decades discovering new ways of bringing denim to high-fashion status.

Like Goldschmied, he spends hours a day at the washhouse, perfecting new techniques and checking in on the product, which is all distressed by hand. Even the leather tags sewn on the back waistband of each pair of jeans are hand stained to achieve the right shade of brown, with a perfectly worn-in feel.

Leave it to LA to bring a traditionally inexpensive work-wear staple like denim and elevate it to a hand-finished product that gleans as much attention as a designer bag. Denim might read as simple and casual to some, but in LA it's brimming with possibility, a blank canvas that begs for the intertwined accessories and colorful layers common to the city.

"LA will always be my spiritual home and I look back at my years spent there very fondly," says Phillip Lim, who was raised in Southern California and designed the LA-based line Development before moving to New York and creating his supersuccessful brand of men's and women's clothing and accessories under the 3.1 Phillip Lim label. "I think I would be lying if I said my designs weren't influenced by the LA attitude toward life and the free-spirited, easy way that only really exists there. There is something about the LA state of mind that will always exist in my designs."

Whether designers are locals who began their careers in Los Angeles or just visit

CHARLOTTE RONSON

LA girls know how to put themselves together effortlessly. Their style makes you want to look like you're not trying too hard. LA details are all about mixing it up, like friendship bracelets mixed with Cartier love bracelets or a vintage dress with a hoodie and a Balenciaga bag. The girls can still be luxe but they downplay it with hippie chic.

frequently for inspiration (courtesy of a fruitful vintage excursion or two), the city is teeming with resources for creative minds seeking a spark. And like Lim, many designers inject a casual sensibility into each collection, creating pieces that make sense within the LA lifestyle and beyond.

"It's really hard to live in LA and not be inspired by the landscape and weather," says designer of vividly hued clothing, accessories, and home objects, Trina Turk. "I'm an architectural hobbyist and LA has so much amazing architecture. It's something that has seeped into the sensibility of my brand. Southern California has also been a huge influence on the prints in my line; they have an organic feeling to them—related to the plants and what grows here, like vibrant colored flowers and succulents."

The light in Southern California is also unique to the area and often evokes a dreamy sensibility in collections conceived here.

"As a kid I spent a lot of time at the beach," says Turk. "There's that golden hour where everything looks great and everyone looks great. The blue sky turns to pink then to orange. I always go back to those colors."

While Turk's line is full of vibrant colors and bold patterns that reflect Los Angeles's retro sensibilities, designer Monique Lhuillier works the inspiration she absorbs from the city into her elegant bridal collection and line of sophisticated cocktail dresses.

"Living in Los Angeles has had a great impact on my work," she says. "I am inspired by my beautiful surroundings, interesting and diverse groups of people, and an incredible art scene." She adds that even though her pieces cater to more dressed-up occasions, she consistently imbues her collections with a chic West Coast ease.

And really, how could LA's climate, size, comparatively laid-back culture, and celebrity influence not create the perfect storm for looks that end up inspiring fashion on a global scale? The casual chic nature that embodies LA-style today is infectious for its deliberate eye toward current trends and the allure of high fashion, tinged with a down-to-earth appeal that ultimately makes getting dressed effortless, personal, and uncomplicated.

STACY BENDET, ALICE + OLIVIA

The LA lifestyle sets a pace for how girls dress. Style is more casual; it has to look good and sexy and doesn't have to be too formal.

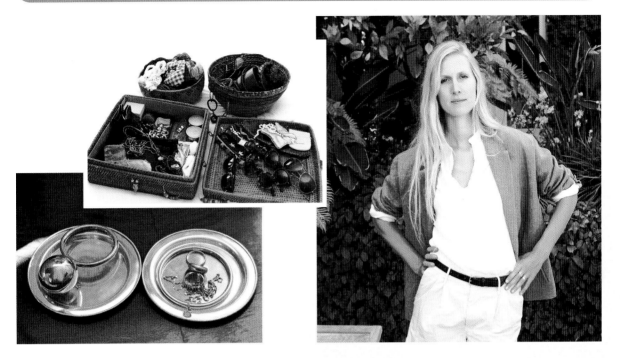

Name: **JESSICA DE RUITER**   Hometown: TORONTO, CANADA   Occupation: STYLIST

How would you describe your style?

Beyond the urgency of fashion. My style is more classic and possesses a simple sophistication. I also believe that true style is not just in the way one dresses. It encompasses the way one chooses to live their life. It can extend to the way one decorates their home, cooks, how one entertains and treats others.

Who are your style icons?

My mother has always been a huge inspiration to me. She has a very timeless style and innate grace. Lauren Hutton is an icon for me as well. Both are examples of classic, natural, sexy, strong women who really look stunning in a men's shirt . . . and both were models too, which helps!

Do you have any items you wear daily or almost daily?

Definitely. I am always drawn to sharp pencil skirts, men's button-down shirts, white jeans, well-tailored jackets, and narrow pants cropped just above the ankle. And I love brown leather belts and treasure plain yellow gold jewelry given to me by family. I have two of my mother's old Ralph Lauren belts from the 1980s, which are perfectly worn in and go with almost anything. And a beat-up leather attaché that belonged to my husband's mother is a prize possession that I use for work almost every day.

Who are your favorite designers?

Isabel Marant, Stella McCartney, Chloé, Ralph Lauren, vintage Levi's.

What is your signature hairstyle?

I have always had very long blond hair and I think sometimes it takes on an identity of its own to the point where people know my hair before they know me! I like to wear it very natural and sun-kissed, and I never brush it.

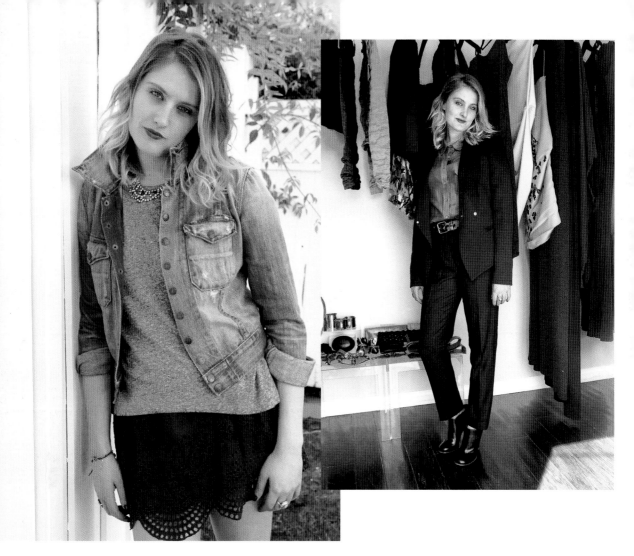

Name: **RENATA FAIMAN**   **Hometown:** LOS ANGELES, CA
Occupation: SENIOR PUBLIC RELATIONS MANAGER

How would you describe your style?

Classic and effortless: I take cues from trends happening in fashion, but it all depends on how I feel and what mood I'm in.

Who are your style icons?

Jane Birkin. I love that French tomboy chic look. I look to European women in general—Parisian women especially. They are just so chic. I love British and French *Vogue*.

What are your favorite items in your closet? And what would you consider a signature aspect of your style?

My Helmut Lang black blazer, Kova &

T party dresses, any striped T-shirts, trouser-style pants. The 1960s are my current decade. I love refined 60s classics.

Who are your favorite designers?

Dries Van Noten, Kova & T, Helmut Lang, Vanessa Bruno, Isabel Marant, APC, Yigal Azrouel and J. Crew.

Do you have any items you wear daily or almost daily?

My vintage ring that's square with diamonds, my oxidized starfish earrings from Garland, and my evil eye bracelet from Israel—I wear these things every day.

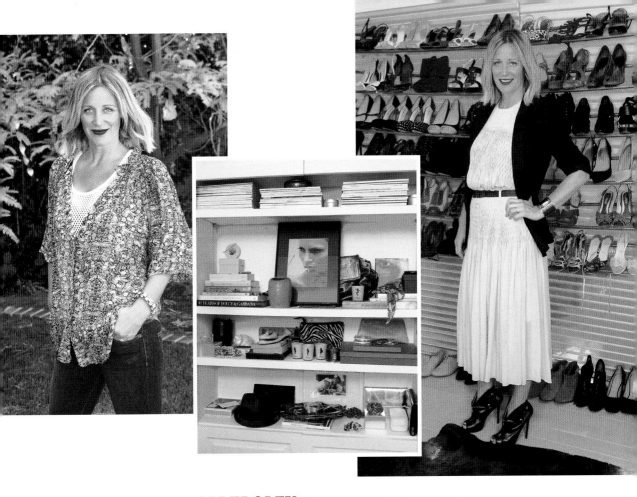

Name: ALI FROLEY   **Hometown:** Danville, CA
Occupation: Fashion Public Relations Director

How would you describe your style?

I'm a Gemini, so my many changing moods inspire me. I don't have a uniform, but I also don't follow every trend out there.

What inspires how you dress? Who are your style icons?

I know what works on me and what doesn't, so I try to follow the flattery rule first and foremost (in that whatever I'm wearing better be flattering). If I had to pick an actual person whose style I admire, it would be Lou Doillon.

What would you consider a signature aspect of your style?

Two items that remain constantly constant in my wardrobe are dresses and high heels. I only wear knee-length dresses or longer. They suit me best. I always love a long-sleeved dress, and a long-sleeve floor-length dress with some kind of fitted waist, preferably in a light silk. I almost never wear flats, unless I'm exercising or at the beach. The higher the better—I like being supertall and, honestly, heels just make you look better.

What is your must-have piece of clothing right now?

My must-have clothing right now is the perfect long skirt, which still eludes me.

Who are your favorite designers?

Dries Van Noten, Isabel Marant, Proenza Schouler, Preen, and Suno.

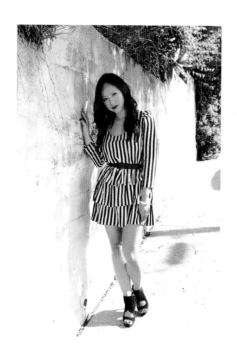
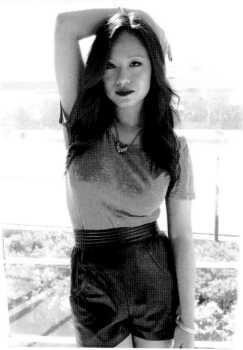

Name: **CHRISTINA TANG** Hometown: LOS ANGELES, CA
Occupation: CREATIVE DIRECTOR

How would you describe your style?
Breezy, subtle, with a mix of edgy and classic.

Who inspires you to get dressed and shop? Who are your style icons?
My friends definitely inspire me the most. I love their personal style and individual quirks. Also, Françoise Hardy, Faye Dunaway, Audrey Hepburn, and Lauren Hutton.

What are your favorite movies for style?
My favorite movies in terms of style are really all over the place. I love *Breakfast at Tiffany's* for the classic chic, *Annie Hall* for the quirky menswear, *Breathless* for the French gamine look, *Valley Girl* for the over-the-top 80s looks, *Pretty Woman* for the body-con amazingness, and *Grease* for the Pink Ladies!

What are the go-to items in your closet? And what would you consider a signature aspect of your style?
My go-to pieces are definitely black denim, colorful scarves, and a great blazer. And I never leave the house without my gold jewelry.

Who are your favorite designers?
The greats: Yves Saint Laurent, Chanel, Alexander McQueen. In terms of contemporary designers, I really like what Rag & Bone is doing.

Name your signature scent, hairstyle, hair color, or other things you feel distinguish your style.
I wear Byredo Gypsy Water almost every day. As for my hair, I'm pretty low maintenance. I just leave it down, and typically keep it wavy. I always wear jewelry, specifically rings (I wear my Cartier love band ring every day) and my Chinese jade bracelet, which I never take off because it's actually physically impossible to get it off my wrist.

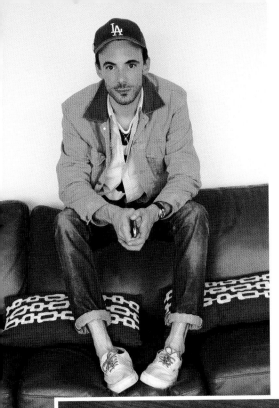

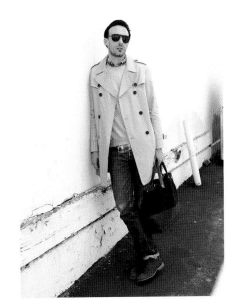

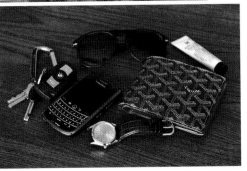

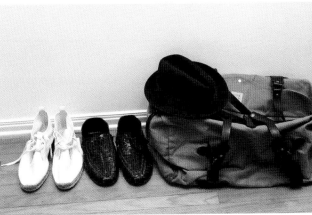

Name: **TODD TOURSO**   Hometown: LOS ANGELES, CA
Occupation: ART DIRECTOR

How would you describe your style?
Italian American via Reseda.

Do you have any style icons or count any films as inspiration?
The 90s and old men, Frank Sinatra, Matthew Williams, and *This Is England*.

What are the go-to pieces in your closet? And what would you consider a signature aspect of your style?
Canvas sneakers, selvage denim, chambray button-ups, and a bad attitude.

What is the last thing you bought?
Vintage Versace 372 sunglasses in black.

Who are your favorite designers and your go-to places to shop?
My favorite designer is Christina Tang and my favorite place to shop is the Rose Bowl Flea Market.

What are your grooming habits? Do you have a signature scent?
My grooming habits are European, or "as needed," Dove soap, and Prada Infusion d'Homme.

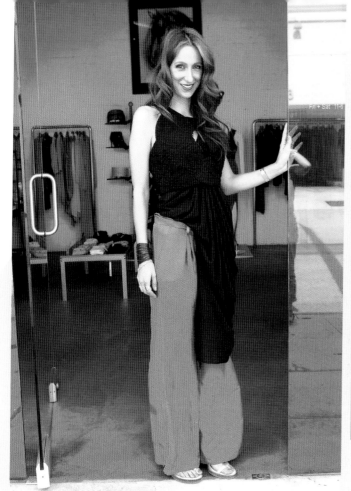

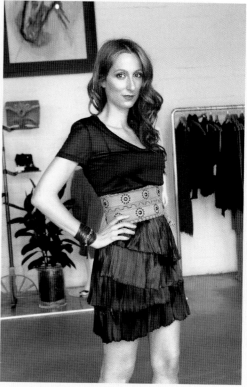

Name: DESIREE KOHAN   Hometown: LOS ANGELES AND MALIBU, CA
Occupation: BOUTIQUE OWNER, BUYER, TREND FORECASTER

How would you describe your style?
Extremely understated. Supersophisticated with attention to detail. Feminine and avant-garde.

Who are your style icons?
I am inspired by street-style. People just walking down the streets whether it is the London streets, Paris fashion week, a private party in Lake Como or in Venice Beach, or a gathering in Topanga. It's always the confident woman who looks effortless in her style—something different that catches my eye.

What are your go-to pieces in your closet?
I have a long pleated Comme des Garçons

skirt that I have been wearing for over ten years. I love that damn skirt and it travels with me everywhere. I almost want to frame it.

What is the last thing you bought? And what is your must-have piece of clothing right now?
My most recent purchase was a vintage kimono. The LA lifestyle is so relaxed that when I am in Malibu I end up wearing long kimonos to the beach and then dressing them up at night.

Who are your favorite designers?
Hussein Chalayan, Juan Carlos Obando, and Azzedine Alaïa.

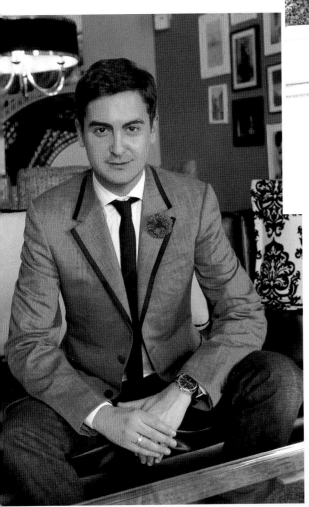

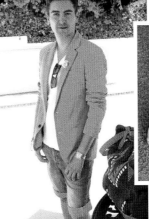

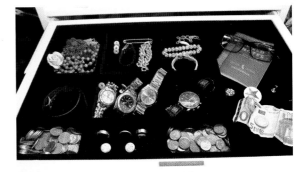

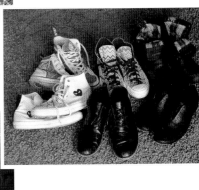

Name: MICAH SCHIFMAN   Hometown: MISSION HILLS, KS
Occupation: FASHION CONSULTANT / PUBLIC RELATIONS

How would you describe your style?
Chill, uniform, understated.

Who or what inspires how you dress? Do you have any style icons or count any films as inspiration?
Other men, sometimes women. Nicolas Ghesquière's personal style.

What are your go-to pieces and/or your favorite item in your closet? And what would you consider a signature aspect of your style?
I'm a denim and blazer guy. I only wear Dior jeans, and blazers by Zara or Lanvin. I also love Lanvin flower pins. They spice up any outfit.

What is the last thing you bought?
Oliver Peoples sunglasses. My rule is to buy a new pair of sunglasses every time daylight savings comes around.

What are your grooming habits? Do you have a signature scent?
I've worn Gendarme for years. It's the best scent—clean and simple.

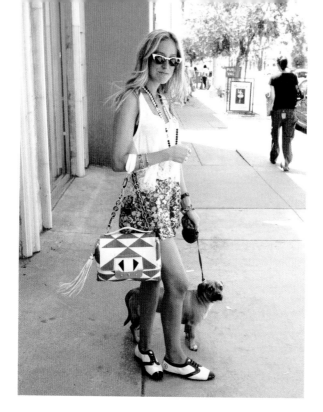

Name: LAUREN "ELSHANE" SHANE   Hometown: LONG ISLAND, NY
Occupation: CELEBRITY STYLIST AND BLOGGER

How would you describe your style?

It's best described as stepping into Dylan's Candy Bar, filling up your clear plastic baggie with everything sour, sweet, chocolate-covered, candy-coated, and caramel-drizzled. Then dumping the bag out on the floor and sweeping it all into one look. I always say, "Life is greener when it's candy-colored."

Who are your style icons?

Gwen Stefani is my number one style icon. I don't believe in trends and Gwen has proven that style can come from within yourself, as opposed to mirrored off the pages of a weekly gossip magazine.

What are the go-to items in your closet?

Accessories are my go-to's because they create so much noise—literally and figuratively! You can hear me walking from a mile away.

What is the last thing you bought?

A giant eight-pointer deer head from a flea market—I made the dealer throw in a pair of vintage Louis Vuitton printed Chuck Taylor Converse high-tops to seal the deal . . . still not sure which part of the purchase I'm more obsessed with.

Who are your favorite designers?

When I dream: Marchesa, Anna Sui, Emilio Pucci, Missoni, Chanel. When I wake: vintage, Alexander Wang, Jill Stuart, vintage, H&M, DVF, Lizzie Fortunato Jewels, vintage.

What are your grooming habits? Do you have a signature scent?

In a city filled with overflowing blond waves (real and fake), I like to be the real deal. I apply and reapply perfume about ten times a day. I mix and match scents, whatever is in my handbag or within reach.

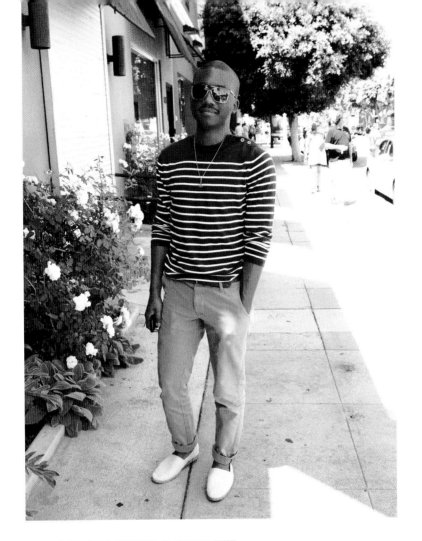

Name: TRAMAYNE LOWREY   Hometown: ORLANDO, FL
Occupation: CORPORATE RECRUITER BY DAY, MUSICIAN BY NIGHT

How would you describe your style?
Urban, fitted, and eclectic.

Do you count any films as style inspiration?
A Streetcar Named Desire, *A Clockwork Orange*, *James Bond*, *North by Northwest*, *Rebel Without a Cause*, *Bullitt*, *American Psycho* . . . (I'm a bit of a film buff).

What is the last thing you bought?
A beautiful pair of blue suede shoes from Zara!

Who are your favorite designers?
Tom Ford, Vincent Flumiani, Dsquared², Barnabe Hardy, Bottega Veneta, Thom Browne, Viktor & Rolf, Phillip Lim to name a few.

Do you have a signature scent?
Tom Ford White Patchouli (which I was told was a unisex fragrance but I believe it may be a woman's fragrance), classic Cartier (Eau de Cartier Concentree), and YSL L'Homme. To me there's nothing more attractive than smelling fantastic!

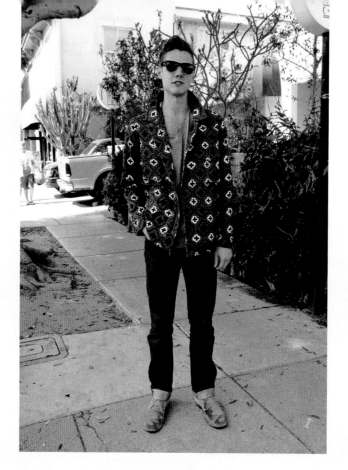

Name: **CHRIS KURSEL**   Hometown: MILWAUKEE, WI
Occupation: VIDEO AND FILM EDITOR

How would you describe your style?
Modern Americana.

Who are your style icons?
Jackson Pollock, David Lynch, my father.

What are your go-to pieces?
Vintage Wrangler denim shirt. Or, when all else fails, a white T-shirt.

What would you consider a signature aspect of your style?
I like contrasting classic simplicity with the slightly bizarre.

What is the last thing you bought?
This jacket (the one in the photograph) and a pair of black boots, both from Opening Ceremony.

Who are your favorite designers?
I don't have one.

What are your grooming habits?
My grooming habits are minimal. The day this photo was taken was the first time I'd shaved with a razor in months. I use Baxter Finley pomade in my hair, or let it go wild.

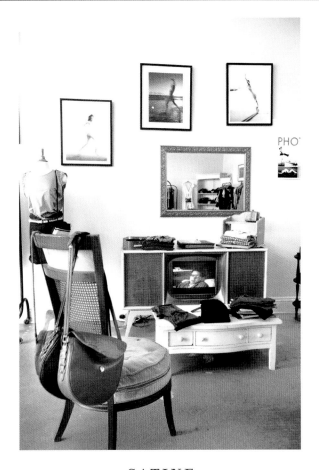

SATINE
8134 W. Third St.
Los Angeles, CA 90048
(323) 655-2142

Nine years ago, Third Street in Los Angeles was a unimpressive stretch of storefronts that boasted established eateries Joan's on Third, Cynthia's, and Doughboys, but not much in the way of chic shopping destinations.

Cut to the summer of 2003, when Jeannie Lee, a lawyer who has always been passionate about fashion and style opened her boutique Satine, which quickly became the go-to location for girls who admired her well-edited selection of Balenciaga heels and Vanessa Bruno blouses. Satine established itself as a source of contemporary and international designer wares and made Third Street a beacon for other retailers to move into the area and create one of the most eclectic and highly trafficked shopping streets in the city.

Lee was attracted to the area initially because of all the independent businesses. "The offbeat mix of stores was important to me because I wanted to capture that indie spirit as well as high-fashion designers and push it through an LA lens," she says. "We're

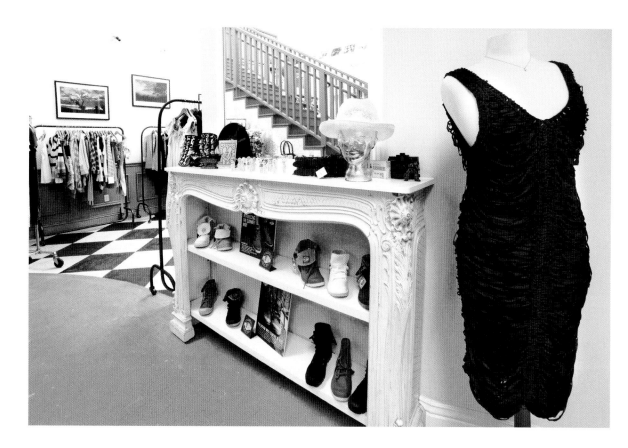

not looking to sell look seventeen straight from the runway. The store, as well as Third Street more than anywhere in the city, is the place where there is a creative, quirky, small business feeling."

Whether sitting in her office or at the front register of the store, Lee is privy to style as it starts on the girls who stroll in sporting everything from Chanel bags and running shorts or their oversize sweaters from their grandfather's closets over a floaty, floral summer frock. Satine is ground zero for the casual chic look at its finest. Girls come in to buy casual chic designer favorites like Isabel Marant and Dries Van Noten and temper them with denim and slouchy trousers.

"We have clients who come in wearing something from Chanel, Zara, or the flea market to their boyfriend's cardigan. This is always how girls in Los Angeles have dressed. They love to raid their grandmother's closets, because there is really cool stuff in there. I see it all before it hits the mainstream. I see these girls create trends."

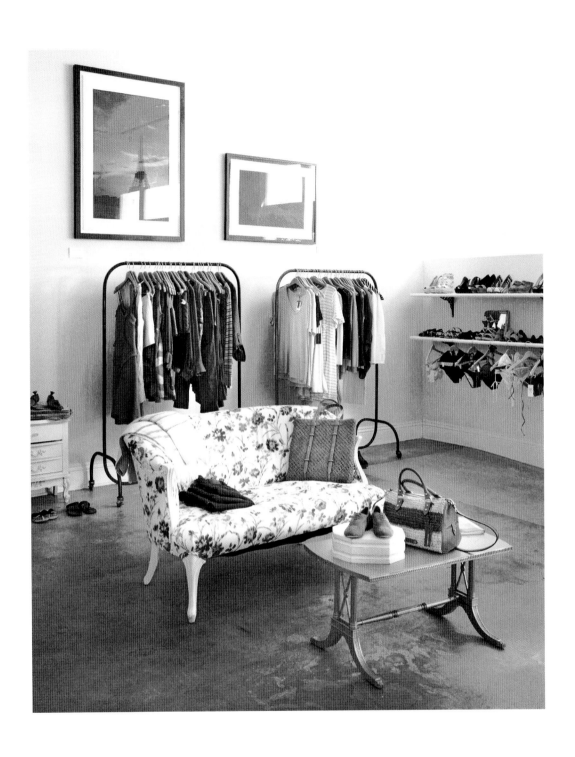

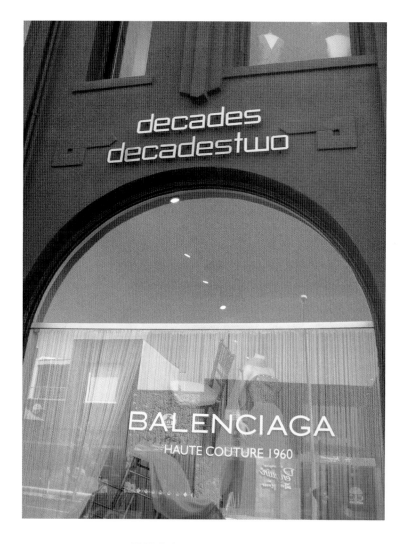

DECADESTWO.1
8214 Melrose Ave.
Los Angeles, CA 90046
(323) 655-1960

If you've ever wondered what it would be like to peek into the closets of some of the most stylish women, celebrities, and taste makers in the world, a trip to DecadesTwo.1 may be as good as it gets. In fact it's better, because here you can actually buy the pieces that once sat in those closets, and for a fraction of the original price.

DecadesTwo.1 is the sister store to Decades and shares a common co-owner in Cameron Silver, who along with Christos Garkinos culls through more than seven thousand pieces of designer ready-to-wear a month sent over from consigners, many of whose high-end wares still have price tags dangling from them. The two opened the store in 1999 after finding that many of the women selling their vintage couture to Silver at Decades had nowhere to bring their contemporary pieces, thus Decades-

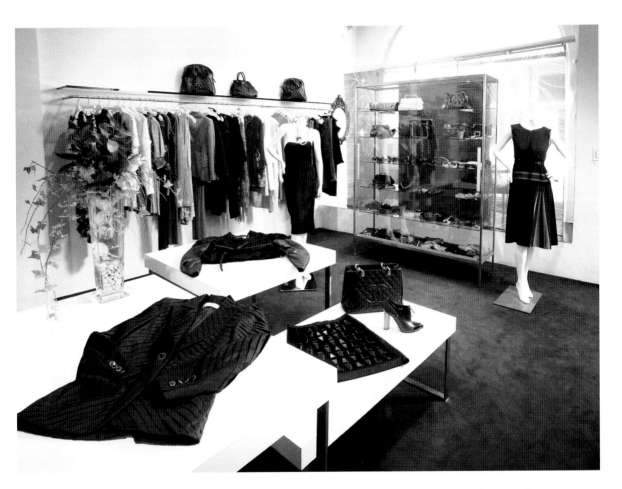

Two.1 was born and it's since been a go-to for trend- and label-conscious girls who effortlessly emulate celebrity-style.

DecadesTwo.1 stocks shelves and racks with accessories and clothing from Chloé, Bottega Veneta, Lanvin, Diane von Furstenberg, Versace, and the most coveted brand among its customers, Chanel. Garkinos claims that most Chanel bags never even hit the floor and there is an arm-long waiting list of women who are ready to pounce once one becomes available.

There are over three thousand consigners who stretch from Beverly Hills to Bahrain and their castoffs aren't just the gain of the average fashion-hungry shopper. Many pieces are picked up by some of the world's most famous fashion designers who drop in from time to time to buy seasons-old pieces for inspiration. Details from the items tend to show up in a collection a year or two later, proving that fashion really is cyclical and DecadesTwo.1 is where trends start, end, and begin again.

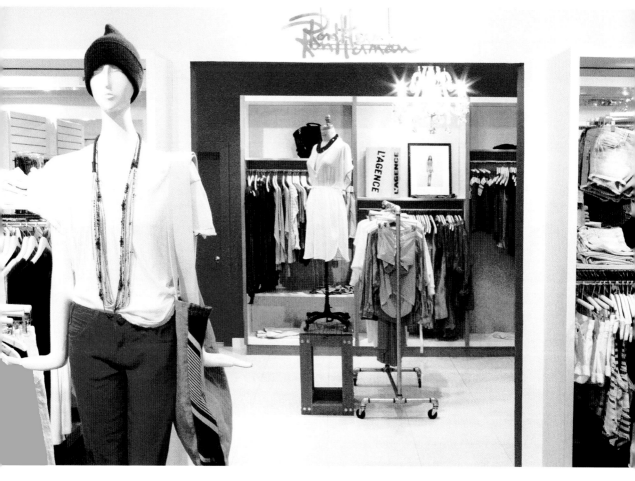

RON HERMAN
8100 Melrose Ave.
Los Angeles, CA 90046
(323) 651-4129

In an era of mass-market fast fashion and sample sale websites, few brick-and-mortar locations remain that can really call themselves a specialty shop. The idea seems somewhat antiquated these days, but it's the specialty retailer with its attention to detail, loyalty to vendors, and unique shopping experience that sets it apart as a classic rather than a relic.

Ron Herman, the women's and men's specialty shop that sits on the corner of Crescent Heights Blvd. and Melrose Avenue,

offers everything from high-end designers to preppy basics and stylish sweatpants. The founder and owner of the store, Ron Herman, has been in business at the West Hollywood location since 1971 and has expanded to three more stores in the LA area, including Beverly Hills, Brentwood, and Malibu, as well as multiple stores in Japan.

Herman's original location is two stories and just over 20,000 square feet of space. To walk through it is to experience the sartorial equivalent of the LA lifestyle, with a sales floor set up to robe someone in all they might need from a day at the beach to a turn on the red carpet. There is a wall of sunglasses from Oliver Peoples, adjacent to a rack of preppy striped shirts and shelves of crochet berets and fedoras. Classic denim from Levi's sits in its own corner section built out to include reclaimed wood shelves and styled to evoke the brand's heritage. It's a prime example of the importance Herman places on merchandising, honoring each brand he sells with its own designated area to really showcase what he sees is special about it.

"A store is a location where we can meet. It's not something that can be duplicated online," says Herman. "The experience is tactile, it's visual, and it has an aspirational value. I remain true to the original idea that people actually enjoy shopping." Herman considers retail a form of entertainment, an escape, and an experience that should be enjoyable. The winding, nook-and-cranny nature of his store certainly lends to the idea of discovery—all with a homey quaintness that somehow makes even high-priced merchandise feel unintimidating.

Herman is selective about everything he stocks, but that doesn't necessarily mean it's all outrageously expensive. There is a section dedicated to a sampling of J. Crew clothing—a brand that he calls exceptional, as well as a room filled with clothing from British retailer Topshop. "This is a comfortable place," says Herman. "You walk in, you see something you like, you touch it, next you try it on, and no matter who you are or what you do, the very last thing you do is buy it. But you do have fun first."

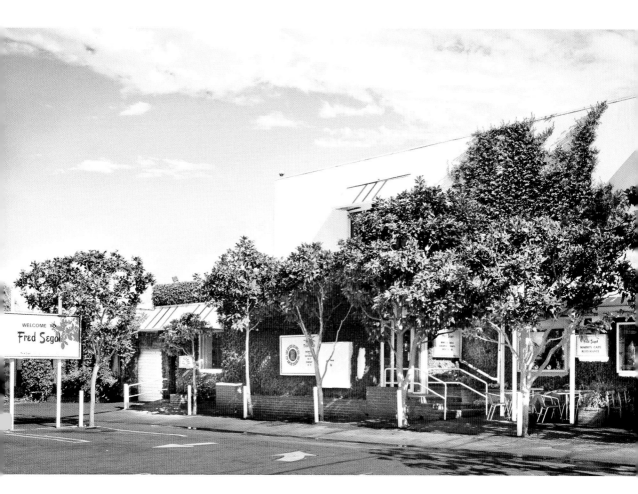

FRED SEGAL

8118 Melrose Ave.
Los Angeles, CA 90046
(323) 651-1800

If there's one store that captures the energy and experience of the LA lifestyle and the casual chic look, it's the sprawling, campuslike retail hub called Fred Segal. The 40,000-square-foot building takes over the southwest corner of Crescent Heights Blvd. and Melrose Avenue and houses hundreds of clothing and accessory lines for women, men, and children, as well as home objects and beauty and fragrance. Call it a quaint department store—or better yet, a hip specialty shop—that focuses on brands suited to the LA climate and a certain level of cool that customers, who include tons of visiting tourists as well as locally based celebrities, have come to expect in the over forty years the store has been in business.

In 1960, Fred Segal, the store's original owner, started with a postage-stamp-sized shop on the same corner and sold only jeans. Segal started a denim frenzy that planted the seed for the premium denim scene that has made LA a center for manufacturing and home to massive jean brands like 7 for All Mankind, Citizens of Humanity, and J Brand. The jeans at Segal's first outpost sold for about $19.95, when the average pair at the time went for closer to $3.00.

The business and physical size of the store grew to encompass more than just denim and catered to the Hollywood set, agents, managers, actors, and overall trend-conscious shoppers who sought out the latest thing. Eventually, Segal began selling areas of the store to key employees to set up their own little shop within a shop, specializing in an area they liked and the unique shopping and retail experience of the multiroom space was born. Each area, no matter whether it's big or small, houses its own focused merchandise—set up and styled to carry out that easy, rambling, and unintimidating sense of discovery.

One of the employees who began working with Segal from the start was Ron Robinson. Robinson started as a salesperson in 1968 and several years later purchased space within the building to open a men's store. Robinson's stores within Fred Segal—simply called Ron Robinson at Fred Segal—take up the second-largest amount of space after the Ron Herman area, which encompasses most of the downstairs area, plus an entire second floor. And though menswear was Robinson's forte, he has since opened a space that sells stylish home objects and books as well as a fragrance and beauty store called Apothia. The store is a haven for any beauty junkie, carrying high-end and harder-to-find goods as well as his own line of fragrance, lotions, and candles.

"This is a boutique specialty shop. It just happens to be larger than most and it's segmented," says Robinson. "It's in its own world. You can come for lunch and shop for shoes and maybe you'll see that hot guy or that hot girl. It's a very big social environment. It becomes that kind of daytime nightclub effect and that's part of a California lifestyle: you can get a cool pair of jeans, a great top, a glass of wine, or maybe you'll see a cool clock that you need for your home."

Also under the Fred Segal roof is a shoe shop as well as luggage and bags rounding out almost every aspect of what a shopper might be looking for—or at the very least providing hours of window-shopping and casual entertainment for customers.

A second Fred Segal store location also exists in Santa Monica, but it's the original store at the corner of Crescent Heights and Melrose that still pulses with history and unmistakable California cool.

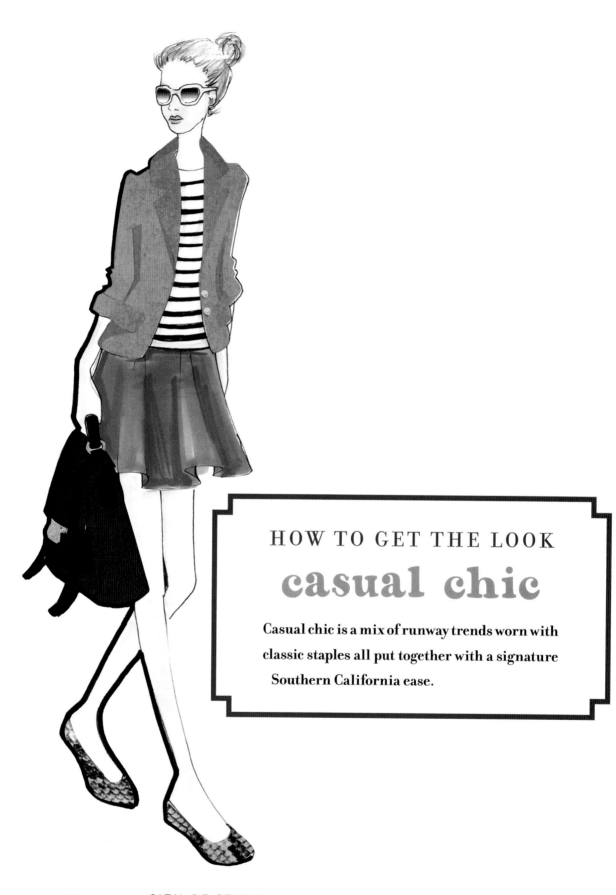

HOW TO GET THE LOOK
casual chic

Casual chic is a mix of runway trends worn with classic staples all put together with a signature Southern California ease.

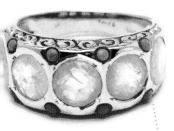

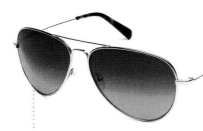

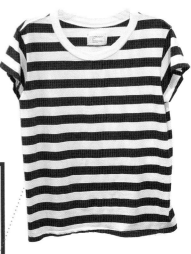

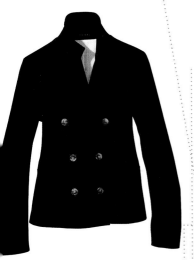

Gold aviator sunglasses are a sleek eyewear staple.

Orange-y red nail lacquer adds a pop of bright color to neutral pieces.

A black blazer is a must, worn over a short belted dress or with cropped jeans.

Trendy accessories like leopard print flats punctuate chic basics.

Rose gold jewelry with a vintage vibe is mixed in with every kind of outfit—dressy or casual.

A striped shirt is a must-have in the high-low mix.

A touch of pink lip gloss adds some easy and effortless shine.

A trendy cross-body bag works from day to night.

Jeans of all styles are at the core of the casual chic look.

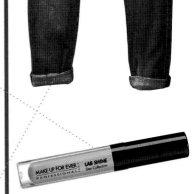

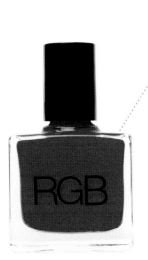

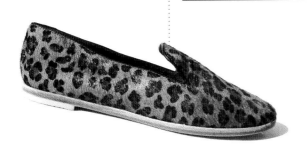

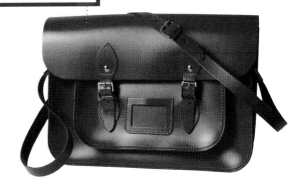

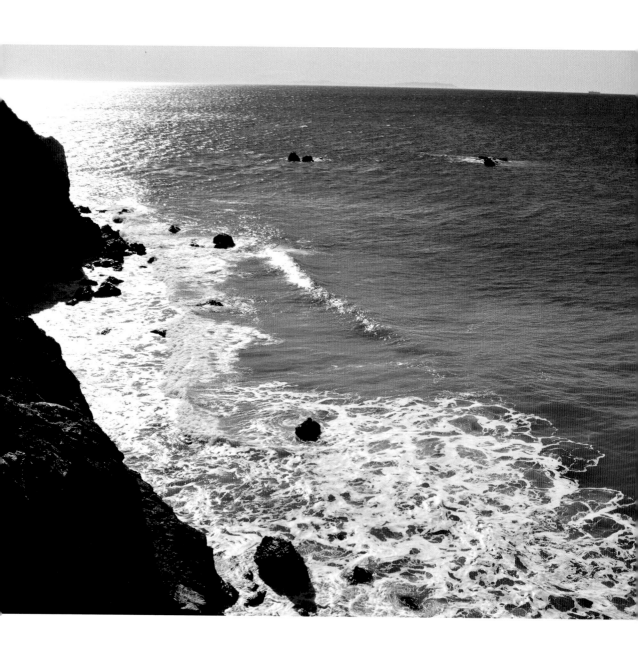

Selected Bibliography

ROMANTIC BOHEMIANS

Kubernik, Harvey, interview with the author, Van Nuys, CA, March 12, 2011.

GLAMOUR

Chierichetti, David, *Hollywood Costume Design* (New York: Crown Publishing Group, 1976).

Cosgrave, Bronwyn, *Made for Each Other* (New York: Bloomsbury USA, 2006).

Engelmeier, Peter W. and Regine, *Fashion in Film* (Munich: Prestel-Verlag, 1990).

Leese, Elizabeth, *Costume Design in the Movies: An Illustrated Guide to the Work of 157 Great Designers* (Mineola, NY: Dover Publications, 1991).

SKATERS AND SURFERS

Kirna Zabete talks surf and sun with Proenza Schouler May 25, 2010, http://fashion.elle.com/blog/2010/05/kirna_zabete_proenza_schouler.html.

CHOLA-STYLE

Cosgrove, Stuart, "The Zoot-Suit and Style Warfare," *Oxford Journals* 18, no. 1 (1984): 77–91.

De Leon, Arnoldo, *Ethnicity in the Sunbelt: A History of Mexican-Americans in Houston* (Houston, TX: University of Houston Mexican American Studies Program, 2001).

Mazon, Mauricio, *The Zoot-Suit Riots: The Psychology of Symbolic Annihilation* (Austin, TX: University of Texas Press, 1984).

Sandoval, Denise, professor of Chicano Studies at California State University–Northridge, interview with the author, California State University–Northridge, January 20, 2011.

Vigil, James Diego, *Barrio Gangs: Street Life and Identity in Southern California* (Austin, TX: University of Texas Press, 1988).

INDIE ECLECTIC

Landis, Dr. Deborah, telephone interview with the author, July 8, 2011.

Maynard, John Arthur, *Venice West: The Beat Generation in Southern California* (New Brunswick, NJ: Rutgers University Press, 1991).

Norton, Sally, "Fashion and Non-fashion and the Beat Generation," gbac.org, www.gbacg.org/costume-resources/original/articles/beats_fashion.pdf.

Photography Credits

FOREWORD

Page x: Amber Valletta attends the Natural Resources Defense Council's Ocean Initiative benefit, hosted By Chanel on June 4, 2011 in Malibu, California. (Photo by Jeffrey Mayer/WireImage)

Chapter 1 ROMANTIC BOHEMIANS

Page xvi, clockwise from top left:

Trina Robbins with Donovan and friends at The Trip, c. 1965, Los Angeles, CA, courtesy of Trina Robbins.

Nurit Wilde, c. 1966, photographed by Henry Diltz, Los Angeles, CA, courtesy of Henry Diltz.

Joni Mitchell seated for a shoot for *Vogue*, November 1968. (Photo by Jack Robinson/Hulton Archive/ Getty Images)

Mary Kate Olsen and Ashley Olsen attend the 32nd Annual AAFA American Image Awards at the Grand Hyatt Hotel on May 26, 2010, in New York City. (Randy Brooke/ WireImage)

Nicole Richie arrives at Beverly Center Fashion's Night Out 2011 on September 8, 2011, in Los Angeles, CA. (Photo by Noel Vasquez/Getty Images)

Actress Angela Lindvall attends Chanel's benefit dinner for the Natural Resources Defense Council's Ocean Initiative at the home of Ron and Kelly Meyer on June 4, 2011, in Malibu, CA. (Photo by David Livingston/Getty Images)

Page 7: Liz Carey photographed in Los Angeles, CA, January 2011, by Donato Sardella.

Page 8: Ronit Nabi photographed in Hollywood, CA, January 2011, by Donato Sardella.

Page 9: Wells Butler photographed in West Hollywood, CA, February 2011 by Donato Sardella.

Page 10: Carrie Jardine photographed in Venice, CA, May 2011, by Donato Sardella.

Page 11: Baelyn Elspeth photographed in Venice, CA, February 2011, by Donato Sardella.

Page 12: Emily Cadenhead photographed in Los Angeles, CA, June 2011 by Donato Sardella.

Page 13: Erin Kincaid photographed in Los Angeles, CA, August 2011, by Donato Sardella. Miwa Sakamoto photographed in Los Angeles, CA, August 2011, by Donato Sardella.

Pages 14 and 15: Enaia Gerber and Johnique Shackelford photographed in Los Angeles, CA, October 2011, by Donato Sardella.

Page 16: Hidden Treasures photographed by Benson Ng for publicityimage.com.

Page 17: Rosebowl Flea Market photographed by Ken Kwok for publicityimage.com

Page 18: Roseark, courtesy of Roseark.

Page 19: Govindas, photographed by Melissa Magsaysay.

Page 21: "How to Get the Look"

Aldo wedge sandal, courtesy of Aldo. Anita Ko Persian turquoise and diamond ring, courtesy of Anita Ko. Joie flower dress and Joie Kadie top, courtesy of Joie. Kangol hat, courtesy of Kangol. Minnetonka Moccasins, courtesy of Minnetonka

Moccasins. Flare leg jeans by Mother Denim, courtesy of Mother Denim. Satya gold bracelet, courtesy of Satya. Scosha NY bracelet, courtesy of Scosha. Simone Camille bag, courtesy of Simone Camille.

Chapter 2 GLAMOUR

Page 22, clockwise from left:

American actress Bette Davis (1908–89) as Madge in the film *Cabin in the Cotton*, directed by Michael Curtiz. (Photo by John Kobal Foundation/Getty Images)

American actress Joan Crawford as she appeared in the title role of Clarence Brown's *Letty Lynton*, wearing a white organdy dress by Adrian, 1932.

Actress Drew Barrymore arrives at the 67th Annual Golden Globe Awards at the Beverly Hilton Hotel on January 17, 2010 in Beverly Hills, CA. (Photo by Jason Merritt/Getty Images)

Portrait of a woman leaning on a wall while modeling a long chiffon dress with a plunging V-neck, ruffled cap sleeves, and a fishtail train, c. 1935. (Photo by Hirz/Getty Images)

Actress Michelle Williams arrives to the 78th Annual Academy Awards at the Kodak Theatre on March 5, 2006, in Hollywood, CA. (Photo by Frazer Harrison/Getty Images)

Actress Diane Kruger at the "Alexander McQueen: Savage Beauty" Costume Institute Gala at the Metropolitan Museum of Art, May 2, 2011, in New York City.

Anne Hathaway attends the 68th Annual Golden Globe Awards at the Beverly Hilton Hotel on January 16, 2011, in Beverly Hills, CA.

Page 29: Shana Honeyman photographed in Burbank, CA, March 2011, by Donato Sardella.

Pages 30 and 31: Sara Riff photographed in Los Angeles, CA, June 2011, by Donato Sardella.

Page 32: Nicole Chavez photographed in Hollywood, CA, April 2011, by Donato Sardella.

Page 33: Cameron Silver photographed in Los Angeles, CA, by Donato Sardella.

Page 34: Rona Stevenson, photographed in Beverly Hills, CA, July 2011, by Donato Sardella.

Page 35: Marc Cireno photographed in Beverly Hills, CA, August 2011, by Donato Sardella. Eri Hoxha photographed in West Hollywood, CA, August 2011, by Donato Sardella.

Page 36: Decades interior, courtesy of Decades.

Page 37: The Way We Wore interior, courtesy of The Way We Wore, photographed by Evans Vestal Ward.

Page 38: Playclothes interior, courtesy of Playclothes, photographed by Julia Dillon.

Page 39: Monique Lhuillier interior, courtesy of Monique Lhuillier.

Page 41: "How to Get the Look"

Jimmy Choo red bag, leopard print scarf, and glitter pump, courtesy of Jimmy Choo. Alice + Olivia fur trimmed vest, courtesy of Alice + Olivia. Anita Ko panther bracelet, courtesy of Anita Ko. Mother Denim black bootcut jeans, courtesy of Mother Denim. Oliver Peoples Racy sunglasses, courtesy of Oliver Peoples. YSL Rouge Couture lipstick, courtesy of YSL. David Meister gown, photographed by Benson Ng for publicityimage.com. Amanda Pearl Rita H clutch, courtesy of Amanda Pearl. Gold sequin top by Alice + Olivia, courtesy of Alice + Olivia.

Chapter 3 SKATERS AND SURFERS

Page 42, clockwise from top:

Hugh Holland, *Sidewalk Surfer*, Huntington Beach, CA, 1976. (Chromogenic print, courtesy of M+B Gallery, Los Angeles)

Model Erin Wasson attends the opening reception at the Opening Ceremony flagship store, Tokyo, August 29, 2009. (Photo by Junko Kimura/Getty Images)

Actress Cameron Diaz prepares to surf on the set of *Charlie's Angels 2*, September 10, 2002, in Malibu, CA. (Photo by Frazer Harrison/Getty Images)

Kate Hudson on vacation in Punta Mita, Mexico, March 10, 2011. (Photo by Christopher Polk/WireImage)

Hayden Panettiere attends Bloomingdale's Santa Monica Surfrider Foundation Celebration Benefit at Bloomingdale's Santa Monica, April 13, 2011. (Photo by Craig Barritt/WireImage)

Page 51: Oleema Kalani Miller photographed in Corona del Mar, CA, April 2011, by Donato Sardella.

Page 52: Kalani Miller photographed in Corona del Mar, CA, April 2011, by Donato Sardella.

Page 53: John Moore photographed in Culver City, CA, May 2011, by Donato Sardella.

Page 54: Alexandra Cassaniti photographed in Venice, CA, May 2011, by Donato Sardella.

Page 55: Lisa Priolo photographed in Venice, CA, June 2011, by Donato Sardella.

Page 56: Cameron Laing, Wade Osborn, and Lauren Phillips photographed in Hollywood, CA, August 2011, by Donato Sardella.

Page 57: Simon Mohos and Tonya Papanikolov

photographed in Venice, CA, August 2011, by Donato Sardella.

Page 58: Jourdan A. Davis and Zac Davis photographed in Santa Monica, CA, August 2011, by Donato Sardella.

Page 59: Xander Mozejewski photographed in Los Angeles, CA, October 2011, by Donato Sardella.

Pages 60 and 62: Val Surf photographed by Benson Ng for publicityimage.com.

Pages 63 and 64: Sportie L.A. photographed by Benson Ng for publicityimage.com.

Pages 64 and 65: Rider Shack, courtesy of Rider Shack.

Pages 66 and 67: Yokishop (interior), courtesy of Yokishop.

Page 69: "How to Get the Look"

For All Mankind denim shorts, courtesy of For All Mankind. Nixon watch, courtesy of Nixon. Vans sneaker, courtesy of Vans. Hurley striped T-shirt, courtesy of Hurley. Kiehl's Super Fluid sunblock, courtesy of Kiehl's. Mikoh bikini, courtesy of Mikoh. Theory mesh sweater, courtesy of Theory. Havaiana flip flop, courtesy of Havaiana. Roxy tote bag, courtesy of Roxy. l.a. Eyeworks sunglasses, courtesy of l.a. Eyeworks.

Chapter 4 ROCKERS

Page 70, clockwise from left:

Slash of Guns N' Roses, holding Gibson Les Paul guitar. (Photo by Robert Knight Archive/Redferns)

Juliette Lewis backstage, before performing at the Miami Dolphins vs. Chicago Bears football game, Miami, FL, November 18, 2010. (Photo by Larry Marano/Getty Images)

Joan Jett of the Runaways, Hollywood Blvd. in Los Angeles, CA, 1977 or 1978. (Photo by Brad Elterman/BuzzFoto/FilmMagic)

The Flying Burrito Brothers, Nudie suits hanging up in the A&M studio. (Photo by Jim McCrary/Redferns)

Nancy Wilson of Heart, 1982. (Photo by Chris Walter/WireImage)

Vanessa Hudgens at the UK premiere of *High School Musical 3*, London, October 7, 2008. (Photo by Ferdaus Shamim/WireImage)

Kelly Osbourne at the G-Star RAW Spring/Summer 2011 fashion show, New York City, September 14, 2010. (Photo by Theo Wargo/WireImage)

Page 79: Jesse Jo Stark photographed in Los Angeles, CA, May 2011, by Donato Sardella.

Page 80: Michelle Laine photographed in Los Angeles, CA, May 2011, by Donato Sardella.

Page 81: Irene Urias photographed in downtown Los Angeles, CA, March 2011, by Donato Sardella.

Page 82: Maryam Malakpour photographed (with daughter Sophie) in Los Angeles, CA, June 2011, by Donato Sardella.

Page 83: Yves Berlin photographed in Los Angeles, CA, June 2011, by Donato Sardella.

Page 84: Jacob DeKat and Prince Chenoa photographed August 2011 by Donato Sardella.

Page 85: Daniel James Resch photographed in Hollywood, CA, October 2011, by Donato Sardella.

Page 86: Joseph Holiday and Nalani photographed in Los Angeles, CA, October 2011, by Donato Sardella.

Page 87: Maxfield, courtesy of Maxfield.

Pages 88 and 89: THVM, courtesy of THVM.

Page 90: MAMEG photographed by Melissa Magsaysay.

Page 90: CERRE, courtesy of CERRE.

Page 93: "How to Get the Look"

BB Dakota Gloria bootie, courtesy of BB Dakota. Belle Noel necklace, courtesy of Glamhouse. Vita Fede Attura clutch, courtesy of Vita Fede. Jack Claudia dress, courtesy of Jack. Newbark Python tote bag, courtesy of Newbark. Jimmy Choo patent leather heel, courtesy of Jimmy Choo. Anita Ko spike rings, courtesy of Anita Ko. Oliver Peoples Jack One sunglasses, courtesy of Oliver Peoples. RGB nail polish in Slate, courtesy of RGB. Current/Elliott leopard-print stiletto skinny jeans, courtesy of Current/Elliott. Benefit Cosmetics Bad Gal eyeliner, courtesy of Benefit Cosmetics. 7 For all Mankind black draped shirt, courtesy of 7 For all Mankind.

Chapter 5 CHOLA-STYLE

Page 94, clockwise from top left:

Fergie of the Black Eyed Peas at the 2005 MuchMusic Video Awards, Toronto, Canada. (Photo by Marc Andrew Deley/FilmMagic)

Gwen Stefani during Olympus Fashion Week, New York, NY, Spring 2006. (Photo by Michael Loccisano/FilmMagic)

Kat Von D at a book-signing for *The Tattoo Chronicles* at Barnes & Noble in Kendall, FL, October 30, 2010. (Photo by Alexander Tamargo/Getty Images)

Singer Miley Cyrus performs at the 21st Annual MuchMusic Video Awards, Toronto, Canada, June 20, 2010. (Photo by George Pimentel/WireImage)

"La Sickass Angel Baby," Los Angeles, CA, 1996. (Photo by Estevan Oriol)

Page 101: Photograph of beach by Cory Desrosiers.

Page 102: Dalina Rebollo photographed in Los Angeles, CA, March 2011, by Donato Sardella.

Page 103: Latina Vamp photographed in Azusa, CA, June 2011, by Donato Sardella.

Page 104: Ricky Roadster photographed in Azusa, CA, June 2011, by Donato Sardella.

Page 105: Guillermo Cuevas photographed August 2011, by Cory Desrosiers.

Page 106: Santee Alley, courtesy of LA Fashion District BID staff.

Page 107: El Pachuco/La Pachuca (exterior) photographed by Rakhee Bhatt.

Page 109: Anaheim Indoor Marketplace, courtesy of Anaheim Indoor Marketplace.

Pages 110 and 111: Greenspan's, courtesy of Josh Greenspan.

Page 113: "How to Get the Look"

Belle Noelle gold hoop earrings, courtesy of Belle Noelle. Kangol fedora, courtesy of Kangol. Alternative Apparel white tank top, courtesy of Alternative Apparel. Milani black liquid eyeliner, courtesy of Milani. MAC Cosmetics lipstick in Hang Up, courtesy of MAC Cosmetics. Converse Chuck Taylor high top, courtesy of Converse. Joe's Jeans plaid button-down shirt, courtesy of Jiro Schneider, Joe's Jeans. Virgins, Saints & Angels rosary necklace, courtesy of Virgins, Saints & Angels. Cheap Monday black skinny jeans, courtesy of Cheap Monday.

Chapter 6 INDIE ECLECTIC

Page 114, clockwise from top left:

A melancholy Clara Bow (1905–65) in a satin dress, 1929. (Photo by Don English/John Kobal Foundation/Getty Images)

Actress Zooey Deschanel attends the premiere of Disney's *Winnie the Pooh* at Walt Disney Studios, Burbank, CA, July 10, 2011. (Photo by Jason LaVeris/FilmMagic)

Actress Kirsten Dunst arrives at "MOCA Presents: Envisioned by Artist Doug Aitken," Los Angeles, CA, November 13, 2010. (Photo by Jordan Strauss/WireImage)

Actress Lucille Ball (1911–89) with her husband, Desi Arnaz (1917–86), c. 1950. (Photo by Archive Photos/Getty Images)

Jenny Lewis poses backstage after her performance at the River to River Festival, New York City, July 4, 2009. (Photo by Roger Kisby/Getty Images)

Page 122: Ilaria Urbinati photographed in Silverlake, CA, June 2011, by Donato Sardella.

Page 123: Julie Ling photographed in Silverlake, CA, March 2011, by Donato Sardella.

Page 124: Melissa Coker photographed in Silverlake, CA, May 2011, by Donato Sardella.

Page 125: Erin Barajas photographed in downtown Los Angeles, CA, May 2011, by Donato Sardella.

Page 126: Ashley Balayut photographed in Irvine, CA, June 2011, by Donato Sardella.

Page 127: Mike Vargas photographed in Los Angeles, CA, June 2011, by Donato Sardella.

Page 128: DeAnne Destler photographed in Silverlake, CA, August 2011, by Donato Sardella.

Page 129: Justine Demeaux photographed in Hollywood, CA, August 2011, by Donato Sardella.

Page 130: Eliza Coupe photographed in Silverlake, CA, August 2011, by Donato Sardella.

Page 131: Michelle von Bauer photographed in West Hollywood, CA, October 2011, by Donato Sardella.

Pages 132 and 133: Confederacy (interior and exterior), photographed by Eric Ray Davidson.

Pages 134 and 135: Ten Over Six, photographed by Benson Ng for publicityimage.com.

Pages 136 and 137: Shareen Vintage, photographed by Benson Ng for publicityimage.com.

Page 138: Melrose Trading Post, courtesy of Melrose Trading Post.

Page 141: "How to Get the Look"

OPI Nail Lacquer in Blue My Mind, courtesy of OPI. Aldo brown oxford, courtesy of Aldo. Bird gray blazer, courtesy of Bird. Corey Lynn Calter dress, photographed by Benson Ng/PublicityImage.com. Current/Elliott roller jean, courtesy of Current/Elliott. Mulberry Lily bag in bright cabbage sparkle tweed, courtesy of Mulberry. Garland Collection rose gold nameplate necklace, courtesy of Garland Collection. l.a. Eyeworks Backbeat glasses, courtesy of l.a. Eyeworks. Benefit Cosmetics tinted lip balm, courtesy of Kirk Amyx for Benefit. Equipment blouse, courtesy of Equipment.

Chapter 7 CASUAL CHIC

Page 142, clockwise from left:

Actress Kate Bosworth attends *The King's Speech* awards season party at Chateau Marmont, Los Angeles, CA, on February 7, 2011. (Photo by Jeff Vespa/WireImage)

Lauren Conrad arrives at *Us Weekly*'s 2011 "Hot Hollywood Party," Hollywood, CA, April 26, 2011. (Photo by Jon Kopaloff/FilmMagic)

Nicole Richie attends a Coachella BBQ at the Parker Palm Springs, Palm Springs, CA, April 16, 2011. (Photo by Donato Sardella/WireImage)

Actress Zoe Saldana arrives at Nickelodeon's 23rd Annual Kid's Choice Awards, Los Angeles, CA, March 27, 2010. (Photo by Michael Buckner/Getty Images)

Actress Rachel Bilson departs from Los Angeles International Airport, Los Angeles, CA, May 17, 2010. (Photo by KBX/FilmMagic)

Page 149: Jessica De Ruiter photographed in Los Angeles, CA, June 2011, by Donato Sardella.

Page 150: Renata Faiman photographed in Beverly Hills, CA, February 2011, by Donato Sardella.

Page 151: Ali Froley photographed in Woodland Hills, CA, May 2011, by Donato Sardella.

Page 152: Christina Tang photographed in Los Angeles, CA, May 2011, by Donato Sardella.

Page 153: Todd Tourso photographed in Los Angeles, CA, June 2011, by Donato Sardella.

Page 154: Desiree Kohan photographed in Los Angeles, CA, June 2011, by Donato Sardella.

Page 155: Micah Schifman photographed in West Hollywood, CA, June 2011, by Donato Sardella.

Page 156: Lauren Shane photographed August 2011, by Donato Sardella.

Page 157: Tramayne Lowrey photographed August 2011, by Donato Sardella.

Page 158: Chris Kursel photographed August 2011, by Donato Sardella.

Pages 159, 160, and 161: Satine, photographed by Benson Ng/PublicityImage.com.

Pages 161 and 163: Decadestwo.1, courtesy of Decadestwo.1.

Page 164: Ron Herman, courtesy of Ron Herman.

Page 165: Fred Segal exterior, courtesy of Fred Segal

Page 165: "How to Get the Look"

Current/Elliott stiletto jeans, courtesy of Current/Elliott. Arik Kastan rose gold ring, courtesy of Arik Kastan. Matt Bernson leopard-print loafer, courtesy of Matt Bernson. The Original Satchel Store pillar red satchel, courtesy of Original Satchel Store. Current/Elliott striped T-shirt, courtesy of Current/Elliott. Theory black double-breasted blazer, courtesy of Theory. RGB nail polish in Too Red, courtesy of David Uzzardi/RGB. Salt Optics Vargas Aviator sunglasses, courtesy of Salt Optics. Makeup For Ever Lab Shine lip gloss, courtesy of Makeup For Ever.

Page 170: Photograph of beach by Cory Desrosiers.

Acknowledgments

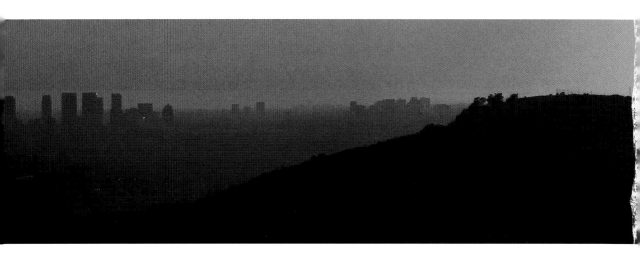

Photographer: Donato Sardella

Photo Editor: Christina M. Pompa-Kwok for PublicityImage.com

Researcher: Erin Weinger

Thank you to the following people:

Donato, you are so talented and wonderful to work with.

Thank you Christina, for your eye, expertise, and dedication.

Erin, you are a super researcher and amazing sounding board.

Ryan D. Harbage, thanks for believing in this from the beginning.

Melissa, thanks for your hard work and gorgeous illustrations.

Emili, thanks for all of the incredible advice and friendship.

Thank you to Jennifer Schuster for your incredible guidance and patience, Carrie Kania, Joseph Papa, and everyone at HarperCollins for their help and support.

Amber Valletta, Harvey Kubernik, Professor Denise Sandoval, Tiffany Caronia, Jennifer Gross, Dr. Richard Schachter, Micah Schifman, Renata Faiman, Melissa Boock, Ali Froley, Collette Pollard, Lori Petermann, Jane Black, Monica Corcoran, Kali Ciesemier, Rakhee Bhatt, Nicole Perna, Marilyn Ruiz, Joey Santos, Alice Short, and Susan Denley.

Photographers Estevan Oriol, Henry Diltz, Hugh Holland, and Benson Ng.

Thank you to all the people who opened up their homes and closets to share their style with us, and all the wonderful musicians, designers, retailers, and stylists who lent their voices and time to this project. To all of the publicists who facilitated my many requests for interviews and images, I appreciate your help.

Thank you Mom, Dad, and Matthew for the constant and colossal amounts of love and support in this endeavor and everything I do.

Cory, thank you for the love and motivation. You make everything possible.